Lecture Notes in Computer Science   7789

Commenced Publication in 1973
Founding and Former Series Editors:
Gerhard Goos, Juris Hartmanis, and Jan van Le~~~

T0177999

Jens Weber   Isabelle Perseil

Foundations of Health Information Engineering and Systems

Second International Symposium, FHIES 2012
Paris, France, August 27-28, 2012
Revised Selected Papers

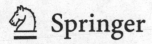 Springer

Volume Editor

Jens Weber
University of Victoria
Faculty of Engineering
Department of Computer Science
Victoria, BC V8W 3P6, Canada
E-mail: jens@uvic.ca

Isabelle Perseil
Inserm
101 rue de Tolbiac
75013 Paris, France
E-mail: isabelle.perseil@inserm.fr

ISSN 0302-9743   e-ISSN 1611-3349
ISBN 978-3-642-39087-6   e-ISBN 978-3-642-39088-3
DOI 10.1007/978-3-642-39088-3
Springer Heidelberg Dordrecht London New York

Library of Congress Control Number: 2013940617

CR Subject Classification (1998): J.3, D.2.4, H.4.1, H.2.7, D.2.11-12, I.6

LNCS Sublibrary: SL 2 – Programming and Software Engineering

Typesetting: Camera-ready by author, data conversion by Scientific Publishing Services, Chennai, India

Printed on acid-free paper

Springer is part of Springer Science+Business Media (www.springer.com)

Preface

Healthcare is among the top challenges for many countries around the world. Industrialized nations face rapidly rising expenditures in light of demographic changes and increasingly expensive and extensive treatment options, while developing nations struggle to improve accessibility to even the most basic healthcare services with a minimum infrastructure and resource support. Information and communication technologies (ICT) are often seen as key enablers for addressing many of the central challenges of today's healthcare environments. Software-intensive devices play an increasingly pivotal role with the potential of making healthcare more efficient and effective.

While some of the expected benefits of these technologies are starting to materialize, our reliance on software for performing increasingly critical functions in healthcare also raises significant risks. Past failures of software-intensive medical devices and resulting technology-induced adverse events have led to increasing calls for dependable quality assurance and certification. Regulators have been mandated to put in place effective certification programs to assure the safety and effectiveness of software in healthcare. Other regulations pertain to informational security and privacy of patients and their caregivers.

One difficulty commonly faced by device manufacturers and regulators is that the foundational body of knowledge for engineering and certifying software-intensive systems in healthcare is not well established. Compared to other industries, the healthcare environment poses several unique challenges that cannot readily be addressed with approaches geared for other critical settings. Moreover, there is a broad spectrum of different types of critical software devices applied in healthcare, ranging from implantable devices, diagnostic and treatment devices at the point of care, to clinical information systems and software-based guideline and decision support (expert) systems.

The symposium series on the Foundations of Health Information Engineering and Systems (FHIES) has been created to provide a venue to foster development and application of theories and methods that can be foundational for modelling, constructing, and certifying high-quality software in support of healthcare. Theories and methods may be adopted and adapted from different disciplines including but not limited to software engineering, systems engineering, data engineering, applied mathematics, and psychology.

This volume contains papers from the second symposium in the FHIES series (FHIES'12), which was held in Paris during August 27–28, 2012, co-located with the 18th International Symposium on Formal Methods. FHIES'12 specifically called for four types of submissions

- Research on how computational models, techniques, and tools of analysis and verification can be applied to problems with software systems in healthcare

- Research on modelling, design, and verification techniques, and innovative practices of software-based ICT and software-intensive medical devices
- Application and integration of foundational methods from different disciplines in engineering and science to software in healthcare
- Foundational research on characterizing and formalizing specific engineering challenges of ICT-based health service delivery in different settings, including developed countries as well as the developing world

Out of 26 submitted papers, the Program Committee (PC) selected 12 full papers and three short papers to be presented at the symposium, following a rigorous review where each paper was refereed by a minimum of three PC members. In addition to the paper presentations, the symposium's program provided for highly interactive sessions with much opportunity for discussion and feedback. Two complementary keynotes by Gerry Douglas and Jacques Grassi and two panel discussions helped to inspire and stimulate the delegates. The authors of presented papers at FHIES'12 were invited to submit revised, extended versions of the papers for possible inclusion in this LNCS volume, taking into account reviewer comments from the pre-symposium review as well as feedback received at the symposium itself. The submitted papers underwent a second round of reviews by the PC prior to acceptance and inclusion in this volume. The accepted papers contain original research results on assuring safety and security in different types of software-based healthcare devices. They cover different phases of the software lifecycle, ranging from requirements engineering to model verification and system certification. They also report and contrast different national perspectives on the topic of development, assurance, and regulation of health software.

We hope that the momentum created during FHIES'12 and the inaugural FHIES'11 symposium in South Africa will continue to grow and propel the next symposium, which is planned to be held in Macau in an expanded, three-day format, hosted by the United Nations University during August 21–23, 2013.

We would like to acknowledge the kind support of the United Nations University's International Institute for Software Technology (IIST). Thanks to the General Chairs Zhiming Lui (UNI-IIST) and Alan Wassyng (McSCert), the Local Organizing Chair Dominique Mery (LORIA), the hard-working members of the PC and their additional reviewers.

January 2013   Jens Weber

Organization

Program Committee

Syed Aljunid	United Nations University - IIGH, Malaysia
Borzoo Bonakdarpour	University of Waterloo, Canada
Stephan Bour	National Institute of Health, USA
Remy Choquet	INSERM, France
Anthony Cleve	University of Namur, Belgium
Christel Daniel	INSERM, France
François Fages	INRIA Rocquencourt, France
Jerome Feret	École Normale Supérieure, France
John Fitzgerald	Newcastle University, UK
Jean-Louis Giavitto	IRCAM, France
Jeremy Gibbons	University of Oxford, UK
David Guiraud	INRIA, France
John Hatcliff	Kansas State University, USA
Mike Hinchey	LERO - University of Limerick, Ireland
Jozef Hooman	Radboud University Nijmegen, The Netherlands
Michaela Huhn	Technische Universität Clausthal, Germany
Henry Kanoui	Ecole Supérieure d'Ingénieurs de Luminy, France
Brian Larson	Kansas State University, USA
Mark Lawford	McMaster University, Canada
Insup Lee	University of Pennsylvania, USA
Martin Leucker	University of Lübeck, Germany
Zhiming Liu	United Nations University - IIST
Wendy MacCaull	St. Francis Xavier University, Canada
Tom Maibaum	McMaster University, Canada
Dominique Mery	Université Henri Poincaré Nancy 1, France
Deshen Moodley	University of KwaZulu-Natal, South Africa
Jun Pang	University of Luxembourg, Luxembourg
Isabelle Perseil	INSERM, France
Anders Ravn	Aalborg University, Denmark
Ita Richardson	LERO - University of Limerick, Ireland
David Robertson	University of Edinburgh, UK
Lutz Schröder	DFKI Bremen and Universität Bremen, Germany
Chris Seebregts	Medical Research Council, South Africa
Kulwinder Singh	University of Calgary, Canada

Neeraj-Kumar Singh	University of York, UK
Oleg Sokolsky	University of Pennsylvania, USA
Michel Sorine	INRIA, Paris-Rocquencourt, France
Alexandre Sztajnberg	UERJ, Brazil
Umit Topaloglu	UAMS, USA
Pieter Van Gorp	Eindhoven University of Technology, The Netherlands
Jens Weber	University of Victoria, Canada
Jim Woodcock	University of York, UK

Additional Reviewers

Chen, Sanjian
Faber, Johannes
Hayman, Jonathan
Ivanov, Radoslav
Jaskolka, Jason
Jiang, Zhihao
Kanaskar, Nitin
Kühn, Franziska

Lee, Insup
Li, Xiaoshan
Meyer, Thomas
Nenov, Yavor
Qamar, Nafees
Roederer, Alex
Schäf, Martin
Wong, Peter

Table of Contents

Modelling and Analysis of Flexible Healthcare Processes Based on Algebraic and Recursive Petri Nets

Awatef Hicheur[1], Amel Ben Dhieb[2], and Kamel Barkaoui[1]

[1] Cedric-Cnam Paris, France
[2] LSITI Enit, Tunis, Tunisia
{awatef.hicheur,kamel.barkaoui}@cnam.fr

Abstract. Healthcare involves distributed and interacting processes which have to be handled in a flexible way due to the variety of individual patient state of health and different kinds of exceptions and deviations that may occur. First, we show how recursive and algebraic workflow Nets (RecWF-Nets) are a promising formalism for modelling and analysis of flexible medical treatment processes where data management and control flow aspects are closely related. Secondly, owing to their semantics defined in terms of generalized rewriting logic, we show that we can check efficiently generic and medical properties of healthcare processes using the Maude LTL model checker.

Keywords: Workflow technology, Distributed and flexible healthcare processes, Recursive and algebraic workflow Nets, LTL Model Checking.

1 Introduction

The recent push for healthcare reform has lead healthcare organizations to reengineer their processes in order to deliver high quality care while at the same time reducing costs and improving their financial assets [6], [10]. For these reasons, the clinical staff tries to optimize patient treatment time in any possible way while keeping the same quality of service by modelling and automating their healthcare processes. Workflow Management Systems (WfMSs) are used in a minority of clinical processes. This is due, in particular, to the fact that healthcare processes (or careflows) are highly unpredictable and extremely dynamic [4], [10], [15], [20] and therefore this poses flexibility requirements on their modelling. Many kinds of exceptions and deviations always occur in clinical processes. Moreover, complex, distributed and interacting processes, with different level of granularity, are often involved in healthcare. Consequently, specifying a real-life healthcare workflow is prone to errors. Incorrectly specified healthcare workflows result in erroneous situations, which may cause disastrous problems in the clinical organisation where they are deployed or more dangerously, on a patient health. Therefore, it is crucial to be able to verify the correctness of a workflow definition before it becomes operational by means of rigorous analysis techniques. For instance, we need to be able to check that a healthcare process always terminates correctly or that contraindications are never administrated. In this paper, we show how we can use Recursive Workflows Nets (abbreviated RecWF-Nets) [4] to model flexible and distributed healthcare processes,

J. Weber and I. Perseil (Eds.): FHIES 2012, LNCS 7789, pp. 1–18, 2013.
© Springer-Verlag Berlin Heidelberg 2013

allowing the users to deviate from the pre-modelled process plan during run-time by offering other alternatives (i.e. creating, deleting or reordering some sub-processes). RecWF-Nets are a sub-class of the Recursive ECATNets [1] which are a special kind of high-level algebraic nets offering a practical *recursive* mechanism for a direct and intuitive support of the dynamic creation, suppression and synchronization of concurrent processes. Furthermore, we show how to check if defined healthcare processes behave correctly before putting them into production. We distinguish two types of properties which must be met by healthcare processes: generic properties related to their control-flow correctness and domain sensitive (medical) properties related to their medical quality and safety requirements [3]. For this purpose, we use the MAUDE system [7] (an implementation system of the rewriting logic [5]) as a simulation environment for the RecWF-nets specifications. In this framework, the LTL (Linear Temporal Logic) Model-Checker tool of MAUDE [24] is used on the RecWF-nets prototypes to check their general and medical sensitive properties. The rest of the paper is organized as follows: In section 2, we discuss flexibility requirements of healthcare workflows. In section 3, we recall the semantics of the Recursive Workflow Nets. In section 4, we illustrate the appropriateness of Recursive Workflow Nets in the healthcare domain through a simple but significant oncology treatment example. In section 5, we show how some properties of healthcare processes can be formally verified using the LTL model-checker of the MAUDE system. In Section 6, we discuss links to related works. Section 7 concludes this paper and provides directions for future studies.

2   Flexibility Requirements of Healthcare Workflows

Workflow models such as those conceived by classic WfMSs are a description of a process of ideal work generally represented in a rigid way [15], [16], [21]. Such representations are not well suited to the reality of organizations where processes are often led to deviate from their initial plans like in healthcare organizations. In fact, healthcare workflows involve coordination of a heterogeneous set of professionals, patients, organizations and sectors and must be able to adapt to inevitable changes of treatment processes, organizational rules [13], environmental conditions and patients requirements. This can be done by opening alternate execution paths, which may not have been foreseen at design-time and not explicitly catered for by the process modelling [20], [12]. This fact challenges traditional WfMSs using an imperative process modelling language such as Business Process Modelling Notation (BPMN) in which the control flow is modelled explicitly. Declarative process languages, allowing any flow that fulfils the specified constraints, have been suggested by a number of researchers as being more appropriate for representing workflow processes requiring a high degree of flexibility [13], [16]. The need for flexible workflow systems and the deployment of standard processes (so called "clinical pathways") [10] seem to be crucial to deliver high-quality services and to reduce staff idle time.

Recently, diverse approaches for enhancing flexibility in workflow processes are proposed where this flexibility requirement is interpreted in different manner, following its application domain [18], [23]. In [18], a set of five distinct approaches are recognized and resumed in the following flexibility patterns:

(1) *Flexibility by design* involves the introduction of advanced modelling constructs into a process model, at design-time, such as cancellation or multiple instantiation of sub-processes.

(2) *Flexibility by underspecification* involves the partial definition of a process model at design-time where the whole structure of some sub-processes will become known only during the execution time by allowing, for example, the late selection or the late modelling of process fragments. (3) *Flexibility by deviation* involves allowing process instances to temporarily deviate from their process definition at runtime, for example, by bypassing or to undoing some tasks. (4) *Flexibility by momentary change* involves changing the structure of a process instance at runtime (for example, by adding or deleting some tasks). (5) *Flexibility by permanent change* involves changing the structure of a process definition at runtime, taking into account the impact of these modifications on all its running process instances (migration instances problem). Based on this referential, an important question to ask is which kind of flexibility is the more adequate for healthcare processes [12], [21], [20]. In this paper, we propose a modelling approach for healthcare processes, based on recursive workflow nets (RecWF-nets), where we focus on design-time flexibility (by design and underspecification). In a first step, these two types of flexibility are sufficient [20] to handle with the required exception mechanisms (e.g. interruption of processes) and the advanced behaviours (e.g. recursion and multiple instantiation of processes) encountered in almost healthcare processes.

3   Recursive Workflow Nets

3.1   Recursive ECATNets Review

Recursive ECATNets (abbreviated RECATNets) [1], [4] are a kind of high level algebraic Petri nets combining the expressive power of abstract data types and Recursive Petri nets [11]. Each RECATNet is associated to an algebraic specification. Each place in such a net is associated to a sort (i.e. a data type of the underlying algebraic specification). A place can contains tokens which are multisets of closed algebraic terms of the same sort of this place. Moreover, transitions are partitioned into two types: *abstract* transitions and *elementary* transitions. Each abstract transition is associated to a *starting marking* represented graphically in a frame.

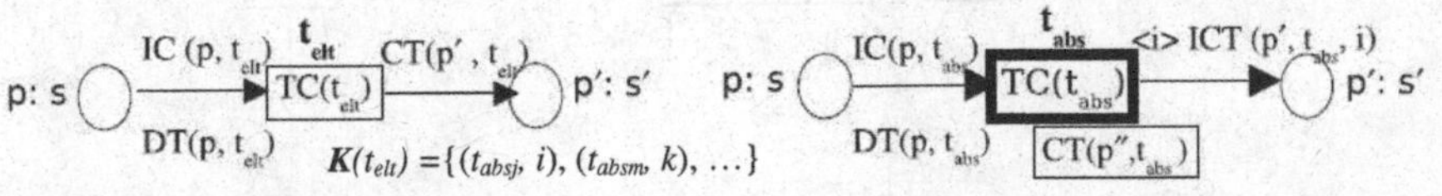

(a) A generic elementary transition   (b) A generic abstract transition

Fig. 1. Transition Types

In a RECATNet, an arc from an input place p to a transition t (elementary or abstract) is labelled by two algebraic expressions $IC(p, t)$ (*Input Condition*) and $DT(p, t)$ (*Destroyed Tokens*). The expression $IC(p, t)$ specifies the partial condition on the marking of the place p for the enabling of t (see table 1). The expression $DT(p, t)$

specifies the multiset of tokens to be removed from the marking of the place *p* when *t* is fired. Also, each transition *t* may be labelled by a Boolean expression *TC(t)* which specifies an additional enabling condition on the values taken by *contextual* variables of *t* (i.e. local variables of the expressions labelling all the input arcs of *t*). When the expression *TC(t)* is omitted, the default value is the term *True*.

Table 1. The different forms of the expression *IC(p, t)* for a given transition *t*

$IC(p, t)$	Enabling condition
α^0	The marking of the place *p* must be equal to α (e.g. $IC(p, t) = \varnothing^0$ means the marking of *p* must be empty).
$\alpha+$	The marking of the place *p* must include α (e.g. $IC(p, t) = \varnothing^+$ means condition is always satisfied).
$\alpha-$	The marking of the place *p* must not include α, with $\alpha \neq \varnothing$.
$\alpha 1 \wedge \alpha 2$	Conditions $\alpha1$ and $\alpha2$ are both true.
$\alpha 1 \vee \alpha 2$	$\alpha1$ or $\alpha2$ is true.

For an elementary transition *t*, an output arc *(t, p′)* connecting this transition *t* to a place *p′* is labelled by the expression *CT(p′, t)* (*Created Tokens*). However, for an abstract transition *t*, an output arc *(t, p′)* is labelled by the expression $< i > ICT(p,' t, i)$ (*Indexed Created Tokens*). These two algebraic expressions specify the multiset of terms created in the output place *p′* when the transition *t* is fired.

Note that in a RECATNet, a capacity associated to a place *p* specifies the number of algebraic terms which can be contained in this place for each element of the sort associated to *p*. In the graphical representation of a RECATNet, if $IC(p, t) =_{def} DT(p, t)$ on an input arc *(p, t)* (i.e. $IC(p, t) = \alpha^+$ and $DT(p, t) = \alpha$), the expression $DT(p, t)$ is omitted on this arc. Fig2 illustrates an example of a RECATNet associated to an underling algebraic specification *SpecRecatnet* (described in Fig. 2) and its unbounded places are of the sort *Data* and *CoupleData*.

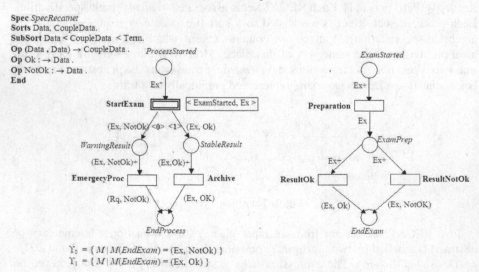

Fig. 2. A RECATNet example

This net has an abstract transition **StartExam** (associated to the starting marking <*ExamStarted,Ex*>), five elementary transitions **Preparation, ResultOk, Archive, ResultNotOk** and **EmergencyProc** and two termination sets $\varUpsilon_0$ and $\varUpsilon_1$.

On the arc (*ProcessStarted, StartExam*), $IC(ProcessStarted, StartExam) = Ex^+$ and $DT(ProcessStarted, StartExam) = Ex$, consequently only the expression Ex^+ is represented in Fig.2.

Informally, the behaviour of a RECATNet can be explained as follows: First, let us note that a particular feature of such net is that there is a clear distinction between the *firing condition* of a given transition t (i.e. condition on the marking of its input place p) and the tokens which may be destroyed from this place p during *the firing action* of t (respectively specified via the expression $IC(p, t)$ and $DT(p, t)$).

Secondly, a RECATNet generates during its execution a dynamical tree of *marked threads* (i.e. sub-processes with an internal marking describing the tokens distribution over their places) called *an extended marking*, which reflects the global state of such net. This latter denotes the fatherhood relation between the generated threads (describing the inter-thread calls). Each of these threads has its own execution context. All threads of such tree can be executed simultaneously independently from each other i.e. a thread can't access to other threads' internal states. A *step* (an *event occurrence*) of a RecWF-net is thus a step of one of its threads. There are three types of events in a RECATNet: the firing of an *abstract transition*, the firing of an *elementary transition* or a *cut step execution*.

The evaluation of the firing conditions of a transition t (elementary or abstract) is always done under a *firing mode* (noted *sub*). A *firing mode is* derived from a consistent *substitution* of the contextual variables of this transition. A transition t is then enabled in a mode *sub* (we say that t is *sub-enabled*) if under this particular variable's substitution, (1) the transition condition $TC(t)$ is evaluated to true and (2) the evaluation of the input condition $IC(p, t)$ of each input arc (p, t) of this transition t is satisfied in the current marking of its input place p and finally (3), the addition of the created tokens to each output place of t must not result in exceeding the capacity of this place when this capacity is finite. So, if a transition t is *sub-enabled* in a thread, it *may fire* in this same mode *sub*. In Fig. 3, we give a firing sequence of the RECATNet of Fig.2, where a black node in the depicted tree of threads denotes the thread in which the following step is fired. For the sake of clarity, each thread is associated to its internal marking, noted in a grey frame.

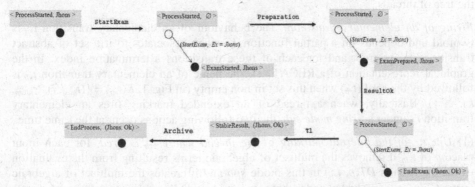

Fig. 3. Firing Sequence of the RECATNet of Fig. 2

Firing of an abstract transition: When a thread of an extended marking fires an abstract transition t_{abs} under a *firing mode sub*, it destroys from each input place p of this transition, the multiset of algebraic terms resulting from the evaluation of the expression $DT(p, t_{abs})$ in this mode *sub*. Simultaneously, it *creates* a new thread (called its child thread and representing a new sub-process) which starts its execution with, as an initial marking, the multiset of terms resulting from the evaluation under the mode *sub* of the starting marking associated to t_{abs}. We note that the fatherhood relationship between these two threads is memorised in the extended marking (we keep track of the name of the abstract transition and the mode of its firing). For instance, in Fig.3, the firing of the abstract transition **StartExam** in the root node of the tree, under the mode (*Ex = Jhons*), generates a new thread with, as a starting marking, a term *Jhons* in the place *ExamStarted*.

Execution of a cut step: The family Υ of final markings associated to a RECATNet is indexed by a finite set of items called *termination indices* (i.e. $\Upsilon = (\Upsilon_i)_{i \in I}$). For instance, in Fig. 2, the termination indices belong to the set $I = \{0, 1\}$. When a thread reaches a final marking belonging to a termination set Υ_i (with $i \in I$), the two following actions occur *simultaneously*: (1) this thread *terminates and aborts* its whole descent of threads. (2) Then, it *produces* (in its father thread) the multiset of algebraic terms in the output places of the abstract transition t_{abs} which gave birth to it. Such a firing is called a *cut step* and is noted τ_i. In this case, the produced terms in each output place p' of this abstract transition t_{abs} result from the evaluation of the expression $ICT(p', t_{abs}, i)$ (where $<i>$ is the termination index of the final marking reached) under the firing mode in which the transition t_{abs} had fired, giving birth to the terminating thread. Therefore, when an abstract transition is fired, the production of tokens in the output places of this transition is delayed until its child thread (i.e. the thread generated by the firing of this transition) terminates and a cut step is executed at this level. Particularly, if a cut step occurs in the root of the tree of threads, it leads to the *empty tree*, noted by $\bot$, from which neither transition nor cut step can occur. In *Fig. 3*, the execution of a cut step τ_i aborts the generated thread (i.e. process) where a final marking is reached (belonging to the termination set Υ_i), reducing the tree of threads to its root process and produces a term (*Jhons, Ok*) in the place *StableResult*.

The produced terms in this place is done using the variable substitution (*Ex = Jhons*), which is the firing mode of the abstract transition **StartExam** memorised in the tree of threads.

Firing of an elementary transition: The behaviour of an elementary transition t_{elt} is twofold and depends on a partial function K which associates to it a set of abstract transitions to interrupt and for each of these transitions a termination index. In the graphical representation of a RECATNet, the name of an elementary transition t_{elt} is followed by the set $K(t_{elt})$ when this set in non empty (in Fig. 1, $K(t_{elt}) = \{(t_{absj}, i), (t_{absm}, k), ...\}$). Basically, when a thread of an extended marking fires an elementary transition t_{elt} under a *firing mode sub*, the two following actions occur at the same time:

(1) *Update of the internal marking of the thread where t_{elt} is fired*: for each input place p of t_{elt}, it removes the multiset of algebraic terms resulting from the evaluation of the expression $DT(p, t_{elt})$ in this mode *sub* and it creates the multiset of algebraic terms $CT(p', t_{elt})$ (evaluated under that same mode *sub*) in each output place p' of t_{elt}.

(2) *Interruption of the threads generated by the abstract transitions associated to* t_{elt}: if the function K is defined for this elementary transition t_{elt}, the firing of this transition performs then the appropriate cut step to each sub-tree generated by the abstract transitions specified by K. So, all threads which are generated by one of the abstract transitions specified by K are aborted and, depending on the termination index associated to it, the output tokens of these abstract transitions are produced in the thread where the firing takes place. In the RECATNet of *Fig 2*, the set K associated to each elementary transition is empty. Consequently, these two elementary transitions update only the internal marking of the thread where they are fired. For instance, in the firing sequence of *Fig. 3*, the firing of the elementary transition (under the mode *Ex = Jhon*) removes the term *Jhon* for its input place *ExamStarted* and produce a term *Jhon* in its output place *ExamPrep*.

3.2 Recursive Workflow Nets

The Recursive Workflow Nets (noted *RecWF-Net)* are a sub-class of the RECATNets model, dedicated to the modelling of flexible and distributed workflows. Consequently, *RecWF-Nets* have structural restrictions which reflect the particular concepts of typical workflows where there is a well-defined starting point and a well-defined ending point. In a *RecWF-Net,* each connected component (i.e, subnet) is called *a workflow component* which specifies the behaviour of a workflow sub-process. A *workflow component* has one source place (i.e. a place without input transitions) and one sink place (i.e. a place without output transitions). Moreover, every place or transition of this subnet is on a directed path from its source to its sink place. In practice, a RecWF-net describes the composition of workflow sub-processes initialised by a principal (i.e. root) process. Let us note that in a RecWF-net, we associate a *finite capacity* to each place connected to an inhibitor arc (i.e. if the input condition on this arc is of the form $IC(p,t)$ $= \alpha^-$). Consequently, interesting properties such as accessibility, boundedness and finiteness remain decidable for RecWF-nets [14]. For instance, the RECATNet depicted in *Fig.2* is an example of a RecWF-net. It describes a simplified process for managing a set of a patient's exams. In this net, we distinguish two workflow components: (1) the component delimited by the source place *ProcessStarted* and the sink place *EndProcess* (representing the *root process*) and (2) the component having the source place *ExamStarted* and the sink place *EndExam.*

   In our compositional modelling approach of flexible healthcare processes we propose to introduce two types of tasks in RecWF-nets: *Elementary tasks* (represented by *elementary* transitions) and *abstract tasks* (represented by *abstract* transitions). The execution of an abstract task dynamically generates a new (lower-level) plan of actions in a workflow process. This plan terminates when it reaches a predicated termination state (a final marking) or when it is interrupted by an exception occurrence in a higher level plan of actions (i.e. by the firing of an elementary transition). In these two cases, the whole descent of action plans, generated by it, are aborted (i.e. a cut step is executed) and the results are returned to the caller abstract task. In fact, a dynamic tree of action plans (with an independent context) describes the structure of a workflow process where all plans can be executed simultaneously. The root plan of such a tree represents the principal process by which the whole specified workflow starts and terminates.

This ability offers the following advantages:

1) Flexibility in workflow planning and execution at design time is introduced naturally. Indeed, RecWF-nets capture the flexibility by design (choice, parallelism, recursion, cancellation and multiple instantiation of processes) and the flexibility by underspecification (*late selection* of process component).

2) Distributed execution of the interacting sub-processes related to healthcare process life-cycle (administrative process, lab testing process, radiology process, care process...etc.) is faithfully reflected.

3) Data and knowledge management of healthcare processes can be easily integrated in RecWF-nets due to state algebraic description.

4   Modelling Chemotherapy Treatment Process Using RecWF-Nets

Based on the characteristics of clinical procedures and medical tasks mentioned in [15], we illustrate the suitability of RecWF-nets in the modelling of a chemotherapy treatment following a breast cancer surgery trough the RecWF-net depicted in *Fig.4* and *Fig.5*.

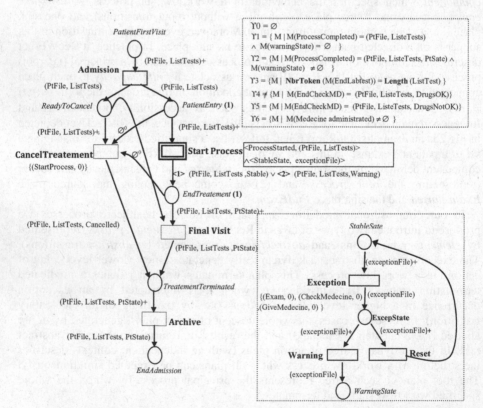

Fig. 4. An example of chemotherapy treatment workflow (part 1)

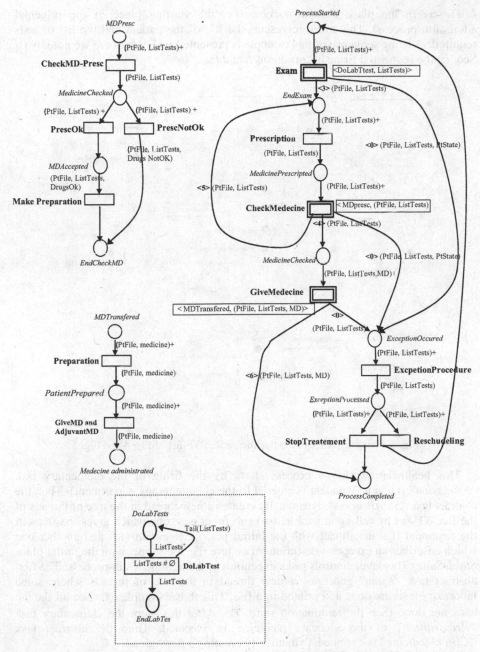

Fig. 5. An example of chemotherapy treatment workflow (part 2)

All the chemotherapy treatment process is based on a flowchart in which basic information about the patient is registered in his file (e.g. weight, height, lab results). All the places of this RecWF-Net are associated to a sort *PatientData*. Let us note that the initial state of this net is a tree containing a single thread with a token (*PtFile,*

ListTests) in the place *PatientFirstVisit* (i.e. the starting place of the principal admission process). This token represents the file of the patient and the list of tests required. A firing sequence of this example is presented in *Fig.6* where we note by (*t₁* Seq. *t₂*) the sequential firing of transitions *t₁* and *t₂*.

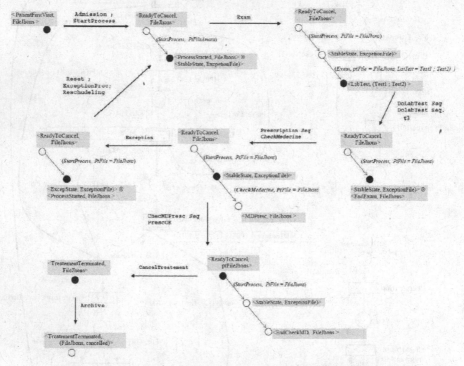

Fig. 6. Firing sequence of the healthcare RecWF-net of Fig. 4 and Fig. 5

This healthcare workflow process starts by the firing of the elementary task *"Admission"* (i.e. a new patient is entered to the chemotherapy department). Then the abstract task *"StartProcess"* dynamically creates a new thread in the tree of threads of the RecWF-net by calling in parallel two sub-processes: one which gives the steps of the treatment (i.e. the subnet with the initial place *ProcessStarted*) and another one which describes an exception detection procedure (i.e. the subnet with the initial place *StableState*).This latter controls tasks execution in the treatment sub-process. The first abstract ·task *"Exam"* generates a new thread in the tree of threads where some laboratory tests are done and printed in a file. This thread completes when all the lab tests are done (See the termination state *Y₃*). After this step, the elementary task *"Prescription"* of the adequate medicine is executed. Then the abstract task *"CheckMedicine"* is executed, dynamically creating a new thread.

Through this new thread, a pharmacy controller checks that drugs dose calculated by the doctor is matched or not with the patient data file (laboratory tests results, measures and adverse effects). The completion of this thread is indicated by a token in the place *EndCheckMD* (See termination states *Y₄* and *Y₅*). If the medicine prescription is not trusted (*Y₅* is reached), a token is created in the place *EndExam* leading to the re-firing of the task *"Prescription"* allowing the assigned doctor to recalculate drug dosages and correct the medicine prescription in the flowchart. If the medicine prescription is trusted (Y_4 is reached), the abstract task *"GiveMedicne"* is fired. In this case, another thread is created in the tree of threads, with the starting marking *<MDTransfered, (ptFile, ListTests, medicine)>*. This new created thread completes when the place *MedecineAdminstrated* is marked (See the final marking Y_6) after what the treatment sub-process completes (the place ProcessCompleted is marked). During the processing of the treatment sub-process, if the elementary transition *"Exception"* is fired (i.e. a medical alert is raised and an exception file is produced), an *interruption* is raised and all the sub-processes produced by the abstract tasks *"Exam"*, *"CheckMedicine"* and *"GiveMedcine"* are stopped and aborted. Note that the elementary transition *"Exception"* interrupts all the threads generated by either the abstract transition *"Exam"*, *"CheckMedicine"* or *"GiveMedcine"* with the termination index <0> (i.e. the list of interrupted abstract transitions associated to this elementary transition is not empty). In this case, a term is produced in the place *ExcepState* and an exception procedure is lunched. After that, depending on the doctor's decision, the treatment sub-process is stopped or rescheduled. Let us note that if the treatment is rescheduled, the exception detection procedure can either be reset to a stable state or ends in a warning state. Depending on the exception file produced, the treatment subprocess terminates in a stable state or in a warning state which has to be watched by future medical procedures (See the termination states Y_1 and Y_2). Finally, at the level of the principal admission process, the doctor supervising the patient treatment has the possibility to stop the whole treatment sub-process along with the exception detection procedure (i.e. the thread is aborted by the firing of the elementary transition *"CancelTreatment"*) as long as the corresponding treatment is not completed. This can happen if the patient decides to leave before the start of the treatment or for another very exceptional reason (e.g. the patient dies). The elementary transition *"CancelTreatment"* interrupts the abstract transition *"StartProcess"* with the termination index <0>. When this transition is fired a term *(ptFile,ListTests, Cancelled)* is produced in the place *TreatementTerminated* but no token is produced in the output place of *StartProcess* (i.e. *ICT(StartProcess, EndTreatement, 0) =∅*). In *Fig.6*, each firing of an abstract transition leads to the creation of a new node in the tree of threads. Also, when a final marking Y_3 is reached in a thread, a cut step τ_5 is executed. The firing of the elementary transition *"Exception"* aborts the thread generated by the abstract transition *"CheckMedecine"*. Then, the exception detection procedure is reset to its stable state and the treatment sub-process is rescheduled. Moreover, the firing of the elementary transition *"CancelTreatement"* aborts the whole treatment sub-process and the exception detection procedure, reducing the tree of threads to its root process with a term *FileJhons* in the place *TreatmentTerminated*.

Such a construction adequately describes the flexible and distributed structure of healthcare workflows where sub-processes may be created or cancelled dynamically (when an exception is raised), leading to rescheduling of some sub-processes. In comparison, modelling cancellation of workflow cases with Coloured Petri Nets would result in net containing spaghetti-like arcs to remove tokens from all combinations of all places [14]. To improve such a modelling, cancellation regions in workflows are often implemented by means of *Reset Nets* [9].

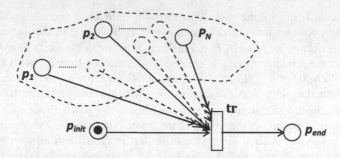

Fig. 7. Modelling a cancellation region with Reset Nets

A Reset Net is a Petri Net with special arcs (called *reset arcs,* represented by a *double headed arrow*), that allow a transition to remove *all* tokens (independently of their number) from its input places when this transition fires. However, the number of reset arcs used in such a modelling depends on the number of places in the cancellation regions of a workflow process (See *Fig. 7*). For instance, in *Fig. 7*, transition *tr* is enabled if and only if there is a token in place p_{init}. After the firing of *tr* all tokens are removed from the places p_1 to p_n and a token is produced in p_{end}. Modelling the cancellation of sub-processes via cut step executions in RecWF-Nets is much more concise because it is independent of the number of places in the aborted processes.

5   Analysis of Healthcare Recursive Workflow Nets

5.1   Correctness Properties of Healthcare RecWF-Nets

With regard to the sensitive nature of a clinical workflow, where human lives are at stake, it is primordial to determine if such a process, based on its definition, behave correctly before its deployment. Testing techniques are not sufficient to prove with confidence the absence of errors in careflow definitions. Testing can find errors but it cannot prove the absence of errors. Therefore, the verification of critical properties of healthcare processes must be done by means of rigorous analysis techniques [3] such as model checking. Model checking is an automatic method which determines if a specified property (formulated in a suitable temporal logic like the Linear Temporal Logic) is satisfied by a description model of a system and its initial state. The model checker will either terminate with the answer true, indicating that the model satisfies the property, or give a counterexample that shows an execution path in which the formula is not satisfied. We distinguish two types of properties in healthcare processes: *generic* properties and *medical* (domain specific) properties [3].

Generic properties specify the control-flow correctness requirements which must be satisfied by every workflow process, regardless of its application domain. For instance, one wants to check (1) if a clinical process can eventually terminate without leaving scheduled or uncompleted tasks, (2) if there is a deadlock or (3) if there is a task which can never be executed. These questions can be resumed into the *soundness* property of a workflow which requires that this latter is always able to terminate properly by reaching its final predicted state and every task of such a process can potentially happen. The soundness of a RECATNet is based on two criteria interpreted on the level of its root process:

1. Proper completion (termination): Starting from an initial extended marking reduced to its root node where only the source place of the principal workflow component is marked, it is always possible to reach a final extended marking reduced to its root node where only the sink place of the principal workflow component is marked.

2. No dead task: In each initially marked workflow component, every transition can fire, at least, once.

Medical properties specify medical constraints and recommendations on healthcare processes, such as relevant clinical parameters or general safety requirements concerning actions of medical staff members [3]. Examples of typical medical properties are: "A patient case must be evaluated by a doctor before beginning treatment", "Contraindications are never administrated" or "A nurse administrates only the medicines given by a doctor".

5.2   RecWF-Net Analysis in the MAUDE System

Since the RecWF-nets semantics is expressed in terms of the generalised rewriting logic [5], [19] each RecWF-net *RN* is defined as a *rewrite theory* $\Re_{RN} = (\Sigma_{RN}, E_{RN}, L_{RN}, R_{RN})$ where the underlying equational theory (Σ_{RN}, E_{RN}) describes the tree structure of its extended marking. Moreover, transitions firing or cut step executions of this net are formally expressed by labelled rewrite rules of the set R (with L the set of their labels). A RecWF-net rewrite rule is of the general form "*Th => Th´ if C*" which means that a fragment of the RecWF-net state fitting pattern *Th* can change to a new local state fitting pattern *Th´*, *concurrently with any other state change*, if the condition *C* holds. Consequently, a *firing sequence* in a RecWF-net is described by a sequence of *concurrent rewritings* in its associated rewrite theory.

Maude is a high-level language [7] and an efficient system based on rewriting logic. The Maude linear temporal logic (LTL) model checker supports on-the-fly explicit-state model checking of concurrent systems expressed as rewrite theories with performance comparable to that of current tools of that kind, such as SPIN [24]. We apply, below, the Maude LTL model checker on recWF-Nets with respect to generic and medical properties.

Generic Properties
1. *Proper termination (Prop$_1$):* This criterion is expressed in LTL by the following formula *Prop1*: **F FinalState** where the proposition *FinalState* is valid in extended marking *Tr* if this latter is reduced to its root process with only one token in its sink place. The temporal operator **F** (*Eventually*) is noted by ⟨ ⟩, in MAUDE notation.
2. *No dead task (Prop$_2$):* We define the parameterised proposition *Excu(t)* which is valid in an extended marking *Tr*, if this transition *t* is enabled in its root node. Thus, to check that there is no dead transitions (transitions which can't fire), we express the

negation of this criterion as the following LTL formula *Prop₂*: $\vee_{t \in Tc}$ (*G* ¬ *Execu(t)*). In this case, such a formula is valid if there is at least one transition is non fireable in the root component of a RecWF-net. The temporal operators *G* (*Globally or always*) and ¬(*not*) are noted, respectively, by [ ] and ~ in MAUDE notation. In the following (see *Fig 8*), we apply the LTL Model-Checker of MAUDE to check these two properties on the RecWF-net of *Fig.4&5*, taking, as an initial state, an extended marking with only a root process and one token (*FileJhons*) in the source place *PatientFirstVisit*. There, we can see that the first property is valid which means the process can always terminate properly. The second property is not valid (a counter-example is returned) which means that there is no transition which is not fireable in the root process of the healthcare RecWFnet. We deduce from these two results, that the healthcare RecWF-net of *Fig.4&5* is *sound*.

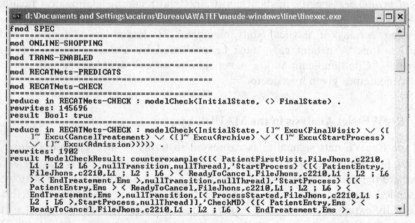

Fig. 8. Verification of the soundness of the RecWF-net (Fig 4&5) using Maude LTL model checker

Medical properties. For instance, for the RecWF-Net of *Fig.4&5*, we use the LTL Maude model checker to check the two following domain specific properties (Fig. 9).

1. *Prop₃*: When an exception is raised, the examination, the treatment and the lab testing processes are stopped which means that all running subprocesses launched by the tasks *Exam*, *CheckMedecine* and *GiveMedecine* are immediately aborted. Such a property is expressed by the following LTL formula where the proposition *RunningSubProcesses* is valid in an extended marking if the thread generated by the abstract task *StarProcess* has at least one subprocess.

G(Enabled(Exception) ∧ *Next(Fired(Exception))* → *Next(¬RuningSubProcesses)).*

2. *Prop₄*: A medicine is administrated to a patient only if it is prescribed by her/his doctor. This property is expressed by the following LTL formula *G(¬(Enabled(Prescription)* ∧ *Next(Excu(Prescription)))* ↦ ¬*(Excu(GiveMD))*)

The temporal operators *Next* and *Leads-to* are noted, respectively, by **o** and | -> in MAUDE notation. In *Fig. 9*, the returned result shows that the properties *Prop₃* and *Prop₄* are true. Let us not that the property *Prop₃* shows the particular feature of recWF-Nets where elementary transitions have the ability to interrupt all the threads generated by several abstract transitions, independently of the number of these threads, in *one step*.

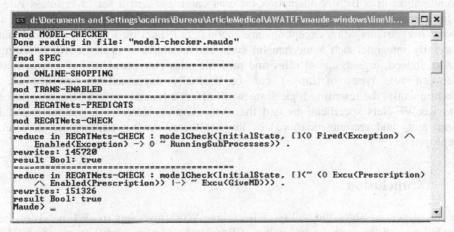

Fig. 9. Verification of two medical properties (*Prop₃* and *Prop₄*) of the RecWF-net (Fig 4&5) using Maude LTL model checker

6   Related Works

Adaptive workflow nets [12] are an instance of the "nets in nets" paradigm, where tokens in a (higher-level) net can be nets themselves. Adaptive workflow nets [12], like RecWF-nets, can change their execution plans by allowing the modelling of the dynamic creation and suppression of processes. However, the advantage of the RecWF-nets is that the distributed execution of workflows and their verification by model checking are intrinsic via the given rewriting semantics. Also, RecWF-nets are more descriptive than Adaptive workflow nets. For instance, in *Fig.5*, when the elementary transition *ExceptionProcedure* is fired, all the running threads, generated by the abstract transitions *Exam*, *CheckMedicine* and *GiveMedicine* are cancelled, independently of their number. Then, the tokens produced in the output places of these abstract transitions depend on the number of the aborted threads. Let us note that the cancellation of these threads and the production of the tokens in the output places of these abstract transitions *happen in one step*. Modelling such a construction is not that direct and simple using Adaptive Nets. In [17], YAWL4Healthcare are introduced to model flexible healthcare processes.

YAWL allows a direct modelling of most complex control-flow structures involving cancellation, multiple instantiation and advanced synchronization, via its predefined constructors. However, the soundness property is not decidable for YAWL specifications where cancellation constructors are used, due to the semantics of the underlying Reset Nets [9]. Consequently, the decision procedures which are developed for the analysis of these YAWL specifications are only partial. In contrast, RecWF-nets allow the modelling of cancellation of sub-processes via cut steps execution while the soundness property remains decidable if their state space is finite.

Finally, BPMN (Business Process Modelling Notation) is widely used to describe the behaviour of clinical workflows [22]. BPMN allows to model cancellation region and compensation actions in such processes. vBPMN framework is defined in [8] as a combination of a BPMN adaptation patterns catalogue and a set of business rules which permit to dynamically activate, on the fly, process fragments creating new workflow variants when exceptions are encountered. In comparison, our model can naturally integrate such a mechanism since its semantics is described in rewriting logic. Indeed, organisational rules and medical rules (for instance, bad interactions between two types of drugs) can be formally expressed as rewrite rules. Consequently, the rewriting logic framework offers a formal unifying framework for the RecWF-Nets specifications and the clinical rules (describing general medical constraints and recommendations) of the healthcare environment where they are deployed.

7   Conclusion

In this paper, we show the ability of Recursive Workflow Nets (recWF-nets) for the modelling and the formal verification of flexible healthcare workflow processes [1], [4]. In future work, we intend to use the temporal extension of recWF-nets, namely, the Temporal Recursive Workflow nets (abbreviated T-RecWF-net) [2] for the modelling and the analysis of real-life healthcare workflows where temporal constraints are preponderant. For instance, it is primordial to specify medical task duration, minimal and maximal time between medicine administration, duration of blood samples or time-out on medical sub-processes. Consequently, time-constrained medical properties in healthcare workflows (e.g. A patient must have been evaluated by a doctor within three weeks before beginning chemotherapy) can be evaluated using the timed LTL model-Checker of MAUDE [7]. Actually, we are working on the implementation of a graphical tool based on rewriting logic (taking MAUDE system as an underlying engine) for creating and analysing recWF-nets. This tool allows edition (via a graphical editor), simulation and verification of recWF-nets using the reachability analysis and the LTL Model checking tools of Maude [24]. Such a tool will propose control flow and flexibility patterns to facilitate workflow modelling.

Limitations. Although, recWFnets are suitable to model and to verify both clinical processes and medical diagnostic protocols, there remains much more to investigate:

1). Healthcare processes entail substantial amounts of concurrency, data and exception handling which lead to very large state spaces. The next step in our work, is to elaborate a more effective analyze procedure for the recWF-nets, to manage the state space explosion problem induced by the reachability graph of huge systems.

In this case, abstraction techniques or hierarchical verification procedures may be adopted. Thanks to the reflective capabilities of the rewriting logic, well supported by the MAUDE system [7] (i.e. the capability to represent rewrite specifications as objects and control their structure and their execution at the meta-level), one can define different rewrite strategies to control the rewriting process in recWF-nets. Such strategies allow, for instance, to partially explore the reachability graph of a recWF-net, in an *hierarchical manner*, for a partial verification of its properties. One can also specify and implement abstraction strategies to reduce the state space of recWF-nets while preserving their interesting properties. In this case these preserved properties are verified by exploring the produced abstraction graphs.

2). reWF-Nets focus on the workflow flexibility requirements which are expressed during build-time (flexibility by *design* and by *underspecification*) [18]. To extend our approach (*flexibility by change*), we can use rewriting strategies to define different structural modification operations on the recWF-Nets specifications to add/change/remove, on the fly, process fragments, places or transitions.

3). We intend also to extend recWF-nets with shared resource concept allowing us to study the efficiency of healthcare workflows taking into account a limited number of available resources (medical staff member and materials).

References

1. Barkaoui, K., Hicheur, A.: Towards Analysis of Flexible and Collaborative. Workflow Using Recursive ECATNets. In: ter Hofstede, A.H.M., Benatallah, B., Paik, H.-Y. (eds.) BPM 2007 Workshops. LNCS, vol. 4928, pp. 232–244. Springer, Heidelberg (2008)
2. Barkaoui, K., Boucheneb, H., Hicheur, A.: Modelling and Analysis of Time-Constrained Flexible Workflows with Time Recursive ECATNets. In: Bruni, R., Wolf, K. (eds.) WS-FM 2008. LNCS, vol. 5387, pp. 19–36. Springer, Heidelberg (2009)
3. Bäumler, S., Balser, M., Dunets, A., Reif, W., Schmitt, J.: Verification of medical guidelines by model checking – a case study. In: Valmari, A. (ed.) SPIN 2006. LNCS, vol. 3925, pp. 219–233. Springer, Heidelberg (2006)
4. Ben Dhieb, A., Barkaoui, K.: On the Modeling of Healthcare Workflows Using Recursive ECATNets. In: Daniel, F., Barkaoui, K., Dustdar, S. (eds.) BPM 2011 Workshops, Part II. LNBIP, vol. 100, pp. 99–107. Springer, Heidelberg (2012)
5. Bruni, R., Meseguer, J.: Semantic foundations for generalized rewrite theories. J. Theor. Comput. Sci. 360(1-3), 386–414 (2006)
6. Cardoen, B., Demeulemeester, E., Beliën, J.: Operating room planning and scheduling: A literature review. European Journal of Operational Research 201(3), 921–932 (2010)
7. Clavel, M., Duran, F., Eker, S., Lincoln, P., Marti-Oliet, N., Meseguer, J., Talcott, J.: Maude Manual (Version 2.3). SRI International and University of Illinois at Urbana-Champaign (2007), http://maude.cs.uiuc.edu/maude2-manual/
8. Döhring, M., Zimmermann, B.: vBPMN: Event-Aware Workflow Variants by Weaving BPMN2 and Business Rules. In: Halpin, T., Nurcan, S., Krogstie, J., Soffer, P., Proper, E., Schmidt, R., Bider, I. (eds.) BPMDS 2011 and EMMSAD 2011. LNBIP, vol. 81, pp. 332–341. Springer, Heidelberg (2011)
9. Dufourd, C., Finkel, A., Schnoebelen, P.: Reset nets between decidability and undecidability. In: Larsen, K.G., Skyum, S., Winskel, G. (eds.) ICALP 1998. LNCS, vol. 1443, pp. 103–115. Springer, Heidelberg (1998)
10. Dadam, P., Reichert, M., Kuhn, K.: Clinical Workflows - The Killer Application for Process-oriented Information Systems? In: Proc. BIS 2000, pp. 36–59 (2000)
11. Haddad, S., Poitrenaud, D.: Recursive Petri nets: Theory and Application to Discrete Event Systems. Acta Informatica 40(7-8), 463–508 (2007)
12. van Hee, K.M., Schonenberg, H., Serebrenik, A., Sidorova, N., van der Werf, J.M.: Adaptive Workflows for Healthcare Information Systems. In: ter Hofstede, A., Benatallah, B., Paik, H.-Y. (eds.) BPM 2007 Workshops. LNCS, vol. 4928, pp. 359–370. Springer, Heidelberg (2008)

13. Hildebrandt, T., Rao Mukkamala, R., Slaats, T.: Declarative Modelling and Safe Distribution of Healthcare Workflows. In: Liu, Z., Wassyng, A. (eds.) FHIES 2011. LNCS, vol. 7151, pp. 39–56. Springer, Heidelberg (2012)
14. Jensen, K.: Coloured Petri Nets. Basic Concepts, Analysis Methods and Practical Use. Monographs in Theoretical Computer Science. Springer (1997)
15. Lenz, R., Reichert, M.U.: IT Support for Healthcare Processes - Premises, Challenges, Perspectives. Data & Knowledge Engineering 61(1), 39–58 (2007)
16. Lyng, K.M., Hildebrandt, T., Mukkamala, R.R.: From paper based clinical practice guidelines to declarative workflow management. In: Ardagna, D., Mecella, M., Yang, J. (eds.) BPM 2008 Workshops. LNBIP, vol. 17, pp. 336–347. Springer, Heidelberg (2009)
17. Mans, R.S., et al.: Supporting healthcare processes with YAWL4Healthcare. In: Ludwig, H., Reijers, H.A. (eds.) Pro: Demo Track of the Nineth Conf. on BPM, pp. 1–6 (2012)
18. Mulyar, N., Russell, N., Van der Aalst, W.M.P.: Process flexibility patterns. Working paper WP 251, Beta Research School (2008)
19. Meseguer, J.: Rewriting Logic as a Semantic Framework for Concurrency. In: Sassone, V., Montanari, U. (eds.) CONCUR 1996. LNCS, vol. 1119, pp. 331–372. Springer, Heidelberg (1996)
20. Reijers, H.A., Russell, N., van der Geer, S., Krekels, G.A.M.: Workflow for Healthcare: A Methodology for Realizing Flexible Medical Treatment Processes. In: Rinderle-Ma, S., Sadiq, S., Leymann, F. (eds.) BPM 2009 Workshops. LNBIP, vol. 43, pp. 593–604. Springer, Heidelberg (2010)
21. Reuter, C., Dadam, P., Rudolph, S., Deiters, W., Trillsch, S.: Guarded Process Spaces (GPS): A Navigation System towards Creation and Dynamic Change of Healthcare Processes from the End-User's Perspective. In: Daniel, F., Barkaoui, K., Dustdar, S. (eds.) BPM 2011 Workshops, Part II. LNBIP, vol. 100, pp. 237–248. Springer, Heidelberg (2012)
22. Richard, M., Rogge-Solti, A.: BPMN for Healthcare Processes. In: Eichhorn, D., Koschmider, A., Zhang, H. (eds.) 3rd Central-European Workshop on Services and their Composition. CEUR Workshop Proceedings, vol. 705, pp. 65–72 (2011)
23. Weber, B., Reichert, M., Rinderle-Ma, S.: Change patterns and change support features– enhancing flexibility in process-aware information systems. Data & Knowledge Engineering 66(3), 438–466 (2008)
24. Ekera, S., Meseguer, J., Sridharanarayananb, A.: The Maude LTL Model Checker. In: Proc. of Rewriting Logic and Its Applications (WRLA 2002). Electronic Notes in Theoretical Computer Science, vol. 71, pp. 162–187 (2002)

Verification of Timed Healthcare Workflows Using Component Timed-Arc Petri Nets

Cristiano Bertolini[1,2], Zhiming Liu[2], and Jiří Srba[3]

[1] Federal University of Pernambuco, Brazil
[2] UNU-IIST, Macau
[3] Aalborg University, Denmark

Abstract. Workflows in modern healthcare systems are becoming increasingly complex and their execution involves concurrency and sharing of resources. The definition, analysis and management of collaborative healthcare workflows requires abstract model notations with a precisely defined semantics and a support for compositional reasoning. We use the formalism of component-based timed-arc Petri Nets (CTAPN) for modular modelling of collaborative healthcare workflows and demonstrate how the model checker TAPAAL supports the verification of their functional and non-functional requirements. To this end, we use CTAPN to define the semantics of the healthcare domain specific graphical notation Little-JIL, extended with timing constrains, and apply it to the case study of blood transfusion. The value added in general, and to Little-JIL in particular, is the formal support for modelling, analysis and verification with the explicit treatment of the timing aspects.

1 Introduction

It is now a global quest to solve the pressing problems of the constantly growing demand with limited resources in providing people with safer, more effective, more patient centered, and more timely, efficient and equitable health systems. The advances in computing and communication technologies provide the potential for solutions by developing integrated health information systems (IHIS) aimed at providing effective support to secure sharing of information and resources across different healthcare settings and collaborative healthcare workflows among different care providers. However, the workflows to provide healthcare within an integrated system become more complex than the traditional sequential processes with standalone systems. Their execution involves concurrency and sharing of resources through synchronization and interaction. They are obviously safety critical, with several non-functional performance prerequisites including timing requirements on top of the functional requirements. Workflow definitions, analysis and management need abstract model notations that have a precisely defined semantics and we need to develop techniques for compositional design and verification in order to ensure their correctness.

Due to the business models and practice of health organizations and healthcare professionals, hospitals and doctors in particular, a rigorous validation and

J. Weber and I. Perseil (Eds.): FHIES 2012, LNCS 7789, pp. 19–36, 2013.

automation of the healthcare processes and workflows are often lacking behind. While formal modelling, validation and automation of general workflows have been an active area of research (see e.g. [6, 22, 25–28]), there has been less work done in the area for healthcare workflows [4,14,18,19,21]. In particular, there is so far only limited effort in the development of healthcare domain specific modelling notations with tool support for workflows. Such a generally accepted notation would form an important step towards the application of formal techniques and tools for modelling and validation in the area of healthcare. According to our knowledge, one of the few established healthcare-domain modelling notations is Little-JIL [29]. It is based on a graphical notation jointly developed by experts in software engineering and healthcare professionals.

There is no formal abstract semantics defined for Little-JIL. Instead, a compiler is developed to translate a Little-JIL model into a finite-state machine (FSM). Simulation of a workflow is done by executing the finite state machine. and properties of a workflow are specified as a property of the state machine, instead of its direct formulation in Little-JIL notation, and FSM-based model checkers can be used for the verification of requirements. The main drawback of Little-JIL semantics (via its associated FMS formalism) is the lack of hierarchy, thus there is no support for modular (compositional) modelling and verification. Furthermore, there is only a limited support for timing in Little-JIL (expressed via durations) and the timing aspects are not reflected in the FSM semantics.

We propose a new semantical approach for Little-JIL workflows based on *Component Timed-Arc Petri Nets* (CTAPNs), a component-based version of Petri nets where timing information is attached to tokens. A CTAPN supports modular specification and verification in general and has an efficient model checker called TAPAAL [9] implementing all the necessary modelling features. In order to demonstrate the suitability of CTAPN for modelling healthcare workflows, we relate it to Little-JIL by showing how to translate the Little-JIL flow primitives into CTAPNs. Our main focus is on the representation of non-functional requirements, mainly the timing; we deliberately stay on a semi-formal level in our translations instead of the fully formal technical treatment that has been already developed for untimed workflows (see e.g. [24] for an overview). We believe that our presentation style will help to highlight the intuition behind the translation, focusing mainly on the timing aspects.

The translation that we present reflects the graphical similarity of CTAPN and Little-JIL notations. CTAPN is a natural choice of our modelling notation also because Petri nets are among the most popular models of workflows in general [11] and because of the available tool support. Compared to the traditional Petri net models of workflows, CTAPNs support a simple and intuitive representation of continuous timing, that is yet expressive enough for describing advanced timing constraints used in workflows. We use the workflow of blood transfusion [8], the benchmarking case study of Little-JIL extended with timing, to illustrate the applicability of our approach.

Related Work. Modelling of workflows using workflow nets is a classical topic (see e.g. [24–27]), however, as timing is becoming a safety critical aspect of healthcare workflows (e.g. blood unit expiration time), extensions of the existing approaches should be studied. For example in [10, 17] the authors study time constrained workflow modelling in the formalism of Time Petri Nets (TPN) [20], a different model than CTAPNs. However, some time requirements like global deadlines, a feature that can be easily modelled in CTAPNs, have to be precomputed [10] due to the missing modelling primitives in the TPN model. Other approaches [19, 21] translate timed YAWL workflows into untimed model checkers via the explicit-time method (clocks are encoded as integers). As advocated by Lamport [16], such methods can compete with real-time model checkers as long as the constants used in the models are small. However, this is not always the case for healthcare workflows—in our case study we used constants of sizes up to 90 and deadlines above 200 minutes with the average size of nonzero constants being 28 (for the model with single patient). The advantage of the CTAPN model and its model checker TAPAAL is that they support real-time verification using the data structure DBM that is less sensitive to the sizes of the constants [16].

Our earlier work [4] proposes to apply the rCOS model-driven method [7, 15] for modelling healthcare workflows, including the blood transfusion case study modelled in CSP. No analysis techniques or tool support are studied in [4]. In the present paper we take the framework one step forward and focus on the modelling of the process view of the workflow with CTAPN and assess the applicability of the verification techniques for CTAPN. Another related work [18, 23] presents a different formal approach for modelling and verification of workflows, including case studies in healthcare. The method and tool is called NOVA. It supports graphical modelling and implements a translation to DiVinE model checker, including timing aspects in the form of delays and durations. The approach considers only discrete time (indirectly simulated in DiVinE) and as remarked in [18], the required verification time is often unacceptable. State-space reduction techniques that include timing aspects are currently under investigation.

Finally, we relate our modelling approach to the domain specific language Little-JIL that already contains a translation into finite-state machines, however, still without the possibility to verify timing aspects. Citing [8]: "Properties B.9 and B.11 involve real time (e.g. an event needs to happen 15 minutes after another event). The current version of FLAVERS and PROPEL does not support real time properties and, thus, we were not able to specify B.9 and B.11 in PROPEL nor check them with FLAVERS." To the best of our knowledge, there is no further published work on tool-supported verification of Little-JIL timing aspects.

2 Blood Transfusion Case Study and Little-JIL

This section gives an informal introduction to the graphical modelling notation of Little-JIL. We will use the blood transfusion workflow for illustration and we start by introducing this case study.

2.1 Blood Transfusion Case Study

We consider the blood transfusion case study from the Little-JIL benchmark [1]. This medical workflow involves a *nurse*, a *doctor*, a *blood bank* and a *patient*; we call them the resources [4]. The patient is required to provide his/her personal details to the nurse. The nurse then carries out the transfusion procedure: (1) the nurse checks the patient's consent with the transfusion; (2) the nurse waits for a doctor to complete the order; (3) the nurse checks the patient's blood type and availability of the blood type in the blood bank; at the same time she books the transfusion room; (4) the blood product is picked up and the transfusion starts; (5) the nurse monitors every 15 minutes the patient and checks for any reaction; (5a) if a reaction occurs, the nurse can try to adjust the IV access; (5b) if there is still a reaction, the nurse must immediately stop the transfusion and informs the doctor; (6) when the transfusion is finished, the transfusion room is released and sterilized and (7) the nurse checks out the patient.

These are only the main steps of the workflow; compensations, exception handling and other details including the timing intervals for all tasks are described in the Little-JIL notation that we shall now introduce.

2.2 Little-JIL

Little-JIL [29] is a visual language used to describe the order and communication between its steps with a particular focus on healthcare workflows. The basic building constructs of Little-JIL are shown in Figure 1. The small circles represent the interface of each activity together with its name and the subactivities are to be interpreted from left to right. In this short overview we represent all Little-JIL primitives in their binary form only[1] and we focus mainly on the flow primitives. Full treatment of the syntax can be found in Little-JIL 1.5 language report [29]. We equip the Little-JIL constructs with more refined timing aspects so that the activities have an execution interval, expressing the uncertainty in the exact duration of the activity, and constructs like iteration allow for time-guarded executions.

A Little-JIL model consists of a finite set of rooted diagrams. Each diagram is either an *atomic activity* (see Figure 1(a)) together with a time interval $[L, U]$ where L is the shortest and U the longest execution time of the activity. Activities can be also exported (calling subactivities specified in separate Little-JIL diagrams) as indicated by the arrow on the external activity presented in Figure 1(b). An activity step can also raise exceptions. In this case a label E: <*exception name*> is displayed below the step box like in Figure 1(c). If the present activity cannot be successfully finished, an exception is raised, the control flow is interrupted, and the exception is passed to the corresponding exception handler. The remaining flow primitives are as follows. Figure 1(d) shows the *choice* constructor. When the choice is activated only one of the sub-steps is executed. Figure 1(e) shows the *parallel* constructor of two steps. In this case all

---

[1] The syntax can be in a straightforward manner extended to multiple subactivites.

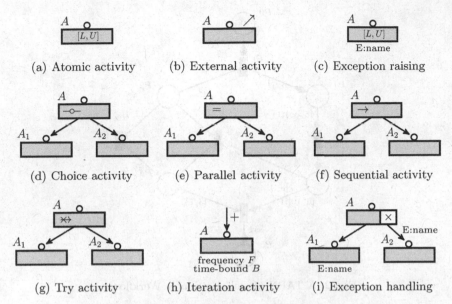

Fig. 1. Little-JIL workflow primitives

sub-steps are executed concurrently and the parallel activity terminates as soon as all its subactivities terminated. Figure 1(f) shows the *sequential* constructor of two steps that are executed sequentially from left to right. Figure 1(g) shows the *try* constructor that allows to try the sub-steps from left to right until one of them succeeds and then the try activity terminates too. Figure 1(h) shows the *iteration* constructor where the activity A is repeatedly executed every F time units until its overall duration reaches the bound B. Then the iteration activity terminates. Figure 1(i) shows the *exception* constructor. The exception handler is also a sub-step but it is specified on the right of the step bar and its scope is for all subactivities, including the exported ones. This is an important feature of Little-JIL since workflows in general handle many exceptions.

3   Modelling of Little-JIL Workflow in TAPN

We shall now introduce component timed-arc Petri nets (CTAPN) and present a compositional translation of Little-JIL constructs into the timed nets.

3.1   Introduction to Component Timed-Arc Petri Nets

Petri nets are a graphical formalism for conceptual modelling of distributed systems. We use a particular real-time extension of Petri nets called Timed-Arc Petri Nets (TAPN) [5,12] where an age (nonnegative real number) is associated to every token in the net and input arcs carry time intervals that restrict the ages of tokens suitable for transition firing.

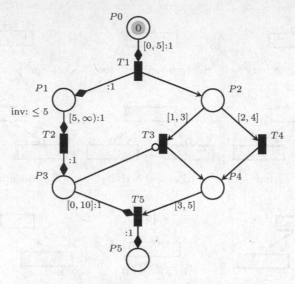

Fig. 2. A TAPN Model of a Simple Workflow

We shall first informally introduce the model. A fully formal treatment of this model can be found e.g. in [13]. Figure 2 shows a simple TAPN model of a workflow process. The net consists of six *places* drawn as circles and five *transitions* drawn as rectangles. The arrows depict different types of *arcs* that connect either places to transitions (input arcs) or transitions to places (output arcs). The dynamics of the net is described by *markings*, i.e. distributions of tokens, each with its own time-stamp (age), in the places of the net. In our example there is one token of age 0 in place $P0$. If tokens of suitable ages are present in all places connected by input arcs to a given transition, the transition gets *enabled* and it can *fire* with the effect of consuming one token of appropriate age from every input place and producing tokens to all places connected with the transition via output arcs. Alternatively, the net can perform a *delay* where all tokens in the net grow older by a given time delay (real number).

In the extended TAPN model we can identify three types of arcs: normal arcs, transport arcs and inhibitor arcs. *Normal arcs* are drawn using a simple arrow tip. Moreover, normal arcs from places to transitions, like the one from place $P2$ to transition $T4$, carry time intervals restricting the ages of tokens that can be consumed by these arcs. Output arcs do not have any associated time interval as the newly produced tokens are by default of age 0. A pair of transitions with diamond-shaped arrow tips, like e.g. from $P0$ to $T1$ and further to $P1$, represent *transport arcs* where the symbol :1 indicates the pairing of input and output transport arcs (in principle there may be several pairs of transport arcs associated with the same transition). The intuition is that once a token is moved along a pair of transport arcs, its age is preserved and not reset. As the whole left-side path from $P0$ to $P5$ consists of only transport arcs, this allows us to measure the total running time of the net since its initialization. Finally, the arc with a circle tip between $P3$ and $T3$ represents an *inhibitor arc*. A presence of at least one token in $P3$ disables the firing of the transition $T3$ but if the place $P3$ is empty then $T3$ is enabled (provided that $P2$ has at least one token of age between 1 and 3) and then the inhibitor arc has no effect on its firing. Notice also that the place $P1$ contains the *age invariant* ≤ 5, meaning that only tokens of age at most 5 are allowed in this place. If there is at least one token of age 5 in $P1$ then no further delay transitions are possible and the net is forced to fire some of its currently enabled transitions.

The workflow net can be executed for example as follows. The first task represented by the transition $T1$ can be performed within the first five time units. If its deadline is missed (which is a valid behaviour of the net) then only time delay transitions are possible and the token in place $P0$ is then called *dead*. Assume that the first task is executed at say 4.5 time units. Then the token of age 4.5 is moved from $P0$ to $P1$ and a new token of age 0 is produced into $P2$. Clearly, none of the transitions is enabled but if we wait 0.5 time units (the maximum allowed time delay due to the age invariant in $P1$) then the transition $T2$ can fire (simulating the execution of the second task) and move the token of age 5 from $P1$ to $P3$. In this particular scenario, the age of the token in $P2$ is now 0.5 and hence no further transitions are currently enabled. However, after say 1.5 time units, $T4$ can fire, leaving us with one token of age 0 in $P4$ and one token of age 6.5 in $P3$. Note that the workflow has in principle a choice between executing the third or fourth task (represented by transitions $T3$ and $T4$), however, in this concrete execution $T3$ is disabled due to the presence of a token in $P3$. After the delay of another 3 time units, the last task represented by $T5$ can be finally executed, producing a token of age 9.5 into the final place $P5$, and the workflow successfully terminates.

During the modelling of larger systems it is often the case that the net becomes too large to provide an effective overview of the structure of the model. In order to overcome this problem, we consider a simple component-based extension of the model. Here we divide the design into a number of smaller components (essentially workflow patterns) with a clearly defined interface in terms of *shared places and transitions*. An example of a Petri net consisting of three components is given in Figure 3. Here the transition T is shared between the components $C1$ and $C2$ and the place P is shared between $C2$ and $C3$. Before the actual analysis of the component-based model, we create a single net by merging the shared places and transitions. This is demonstrated in the lower part of Figure 3.

3.2 Translation of Little-JIL Primitives to CTAPN

We shall now present a translation of Little-JIL workflow constructs extended with explicit timing information into CTAPN. For each Little-JIL activity A we construct a *timed workflow net* (see e.g. [10, 17, 24–27]), a special form of a timed-arc Petri net, where

- there is exactly one *input place* called $start_A$ that has no input arcs, and
- a number of *output places* including end_A and optionally also other places[2] for modelling failed executions and exceptions such that all output places have no outgoing arcs.

---

[2] An extension to the standard workflow nets that only contain one output place.

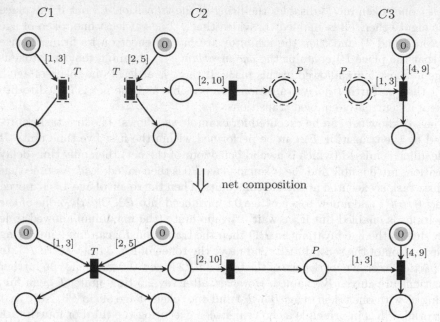

Fig. 3. Components $C1$, $C2$ and $C3$ and the Composed Net

For the external activity call (Figure 1(b)) the input and output places are shared and the activity is modelled in a separate component. In this way the whole net is decomposed into several components that are manageable (usually fit on one screen) and they are composed automatically before the verification of workflow properties is initiated.

We say that a net is *statically sound* if all places and transitions are on a path from the input place to some of the output places. A net is *dynamically sound* if during any execution starting with a marking having a token in the input place, we eventually reach a marking where one of the output places is marked. Note that a statically sound net is not necessarily dynamically sound. We show how to automatically verify dynamical soundness in Section 4. Statical soundness is guaranteed by the compositional construction of the workflow nets.

We say that $[L, U]$, where $L \leq U$, is the *execution interval* of a timed workflow net if L is the shortest and U the longest time needed to move a single token from the input place to some of the output places. Note that if a net is not dynamically sound, the execution interval is not well defined.

We shall now provide the details of the translation for building statically sound workflow nets for the Little-JIL constructs.

Atomic Activity. A timed workflow net corresponding to the atomic activity (Figure 1(a)) is depicted in Figure 4. The presence of the invariant $\leq U$ guarantees that the activity is executed no later than U time units since its initialization and the interval on the arc ensures that this does not happen earlier than at time L. Hence we get the following property.

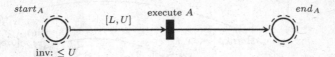

Fig. 4. Atomic activity

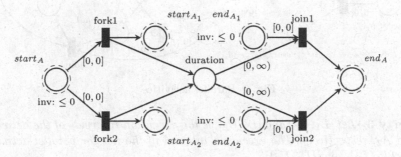

Fig. 5. Alternative activities

Property 1. *The execution interval of the net for atomic activity A is $[L, U]$.*

Note that the input and output places are shared so that they can be composed with other coordinating activities.

Alternative Activities. Figure 5 describes the choice between two alternatives of the Little-JIL diagram in Figure 1(d). The place duration is used to measure the current execution time (represented by the age of a token in this place) of the choice activity. A monitor (see Subsection 3.3) connected to the place duration can be used to detect a possible deadline violation.

Property 2. *Let $[L_1, U_1]$ and $[L_2, U_2]$ be the execution intervals of the activities A_1 and A_2, respectively. The execution interval of the net for alternative activities is $[\min\{L_1, L_2\}, \max\{U_1, U_2\}]$.*

Proof. From the initial marking that contains one token in place $start_A$ we have to, without any further delay due to the invariant ≤ 0, fire either the transition fork1 or fork2. This initiates the subnets for the activity A_1 or A_2. When these are finished, again due to the invariants ≤ 0 in places end_{A_1} and end_{A_2} we have to without any delay fire the transition join1 or join2. The lower and upper bounds of the execution interval are clearly the minimum and the maximum of the corresponding bounds for the activities A_1 and A_2.   □

Parallel Activities. Parallel Little-JIL activities (Figure 1(e)) are modelled by the net in Figure 6. Here the subnets for the activities A_1 and A_2 are initiated concurrently by firing the transition fork. A duration place is added as before for the monitoring of the total duration of the parallel activities. There is added a mechanism that ensures that the place end_A is marked as soon as both parallel subtasks terminate.

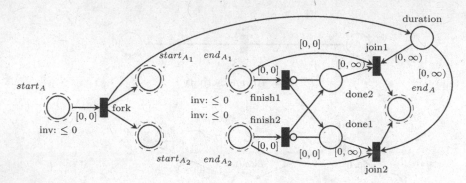

Fig. 6. Parallel activities

Property 3. *Let* $[L_1, U_1]$ *and* $[L_2, U_2]$ *be the execution intervals of the activities* A_1 *and* A_2, *respectively. The execution interval of the net for parallel activities is* $[\max\{L_1, L_2\}, \max\{U_1, U_2\}]$.

Proof. Notice that due to the age invariant ≤ 0 at place $start_A$ the two parallel activities are initiated without any delay. The construction connected to the end states for the two parallel activities ensures that a join happens as soon as both parallel activities mark their output places. Assume w.l.o.g. that the first subnet terminates first and marks the place end_{A_1}. Without further delay (imposed by the invariant ≤ 0 at place end_{A_1}) the transition finish1 must be fired; note that the transition join1 is not enabled. No other transitions are enabled until the subnet for A_2 terminates by placing a token into the place end_{A_2}. In this case the transition finish2 is not enabled due the the inhibitor arc and the fact that done1 already contains a token. Hence, without any further delay, the only option is to fire the transition join2 and mark the output place of the activity net for A (and at the same time consume the token from the place duration). □

Sequential Activities. Figure 7 shows how a diagram A consisting of two sequential Little-JIL activities A_1 and A_2 (described in Figure 1(f)) can be modelled as a timed workflow net. The point is that the first activity is activated immediately and the age of the token in the place duration1 can be used to measure the duration of the first activity. When the first activity is finished, the second activity is initiated without any delay. At the same time the token from duration1 is moved using the transport arcs to the place duration1+2 and its age in this place corresponds to the total duration of the first activity plus the current duration of the second activity. As mentioned before, a monitor can be attached to this place in order to check for the violation of deadlines.

Property 4. *Let* $[L_1, U_1]$ *and* $[L_2, U_2]$ *be the execution intervals of the activities* A_1 *and* A_2, *respectively. The execution interval of the net for sequential activities is* $[L_1 + L_2, U_1 + U_2]$.

Proof. Due to the presence of the invariant ≤ 0 in the place $start_A$, the first activity is initiated without any delay. When it is finished, thanks to the invariant

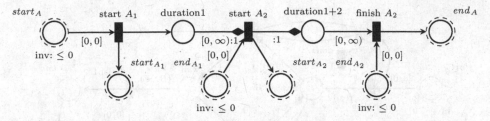

Fig. 7. Sequential activities

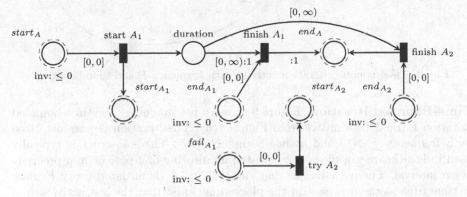

Fig. 8. Try A_1 else execute A_2

≤ 0 in place end_{A_1}, the second activity is initiated without any delay and because of the last invariant ≤ 0 at the place end_{A_2}, the whole workflow finishes in the time corresponding to the sum of the durations of the two activities.   □

Try Activity. In the translation of the try construct (Figure 1(g)) presented in Figure 8, we first start with the execution of the first activity and if it ends successfully the whole try activity ends. If the first activity fails, we execute without any delay the second activity as an alternative. We assume that the net for the first activity A_1 contains a special output place $fail_{A_1}$ that gets marked whenever its execution fails.

Property 5. *Let* $[L_1, U_1]$ *and* $[L_2, U_2]$ *be the execution intervals of the activities* A_1 *and* A_2, *respectively. The execution interval of the net for try activity is* $[L_1, U_1 + U_2]$.

Proof. Clearly the first activity is called without any delay due to the invariant ≤ 0 at the place $start_A$ and within the interval $[L_1, U_1]$ the first subnet marks either end_{A_1} or $fail_{A_1}$. In the first case, again without any delay, the place end_A will be marked; in the second case the second activity is initiated without any delay and the execution of try stops as soon as this activity is finished. Then clearly the shortest execution time is L_1, assuming that the try activity succeeds on the first subactivity, and the longest one is $U_1 + U_2$.   □

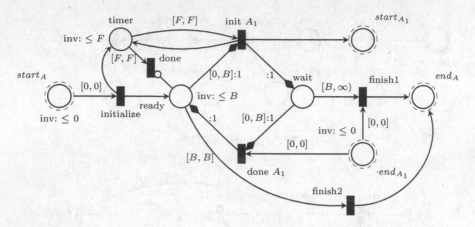

Fig. 9. Time-bounded iteration activity with frequency F and time-bound B

Time-Bounded Iteration. Figure 9 shows a net modelling the time-bounded iteration Little-JIL primitive from Figure 1(h). The iteration is parameterized by a frequency $F > 0$ and a time-bound $B \geq F$. This construct is typically used in healthcare workflows for repeated monitoring of a patient in a precisely given interval. The net enforces that the activity A_1 is initiated every F units of time (due to the invariant in the place timer) and that the last activation of A_1 happens no later then B time units from the activation of the iteration net.

After initializing the net and placing a token into the place ready and into the timer, we delay F time units and start the subactivity A_1. The token from the place ready is moved to the place wait while its age is being preserved; at the same time the age of the token in the timer is reset to zero. Once the activity A_1 is finished, we have to fire (with no delay) the transition done A_1 and move the token from wait to ready (unless the iteration is ended by firing finish1). Thanks to the transport arcs, the age of the token in ready measures the total execution time of the iteration activity.

The reader may observe that if the duration of the activity A_1 is longer than the frequency F then the token in the place timer will be removed by firing the transition done and once the place ready gets marked by firing the transition done A_1, the activation of A_1 at the frequency F is broken. We can detect such a situation via monitors.

Property 6. *Let $[L_1, U_1]$ be the execution interval of the activity A_1. The execution interval of the net for iteration activity is $[B, \max\{B, kF + U_1\}]$ where k is the largest integer such that $kF \leq B$.*

Proof. The lower bound of B time units is easy to prove as the age of the token that it moved by the transport arcs between the places ready and wait corresponds to the total duration of the iteration activity. The workflow can be terminated by firing either the transition finish1 or finish2 and both of them require a token of age at least B.

For the upper bound, we consider two cases. If $U_1 > F$ then during the slowest execution of A_1, the token in the place timer will be consumed and once the place ready gets marked, we can only wait until the total time reaches B and then fire the transition finish2. Hence the upper bound in this case is B.

If $U_1 \leq F$ then the transition init A_1 will be fired regularly after each F time units until the age of the token in the places ready or wait reaches the age B. This means that the last time the transition init A_1 can be fired is at the moment kF where k is the largest integer such that $kF \leq B$. After that we wait for the termination of the execution of A_1. In the worst scenario this takes U_1 time units, so the total execution time is $kF + U_1$ and if this exceeds the bound B then we are forced to fire immediately the transition finish1 and the longest execution time is $kF + U_1$. $\square$

3.3   Additional Workflow Modelling Features

Exception Handling. We handle the exceptions (Figure 1(i)) in a similar way as the try construct presented in Figure 8. An atomic subactivity of A_1 (here not necessarily only a part of the sequential composition) can raise an exception E:name by placing a token into a new output place $exception_{name}$. The exception should be now caught by the first exception handler that covers its scope. As the nesting of exceptions in Little-JIL is always finite, we can create more copies of the place $exception_{name}$, one for each scope of the exception handler. The scopes are then updated dynamically during the computation of the net. As the scope information is finite, it is not surprising that we can remember its scope in this way. Nevertheless it is technically challenging to manually model multiple nested exceptions. In the case study we therefore used only a single nesting of exceptions that is easily manageable for a human modeller.

Shared Resources with Timing. Little-JIL provides also a mechanism for acquiring and releasing resources. Resources with exclusive access can be modelled in Petri nets in the standard way; we add here the additional option to measure the recovery time that has to pass from the time a resource was released until it can be acquired by another process. For example in our case study two nurses need to acquire a room for a transfusion and we have to guarantee exclusive access to the room. Moreover, after the room is released, some other activity (e.g. sterilization) must be performed before the room is ready for another patient. We can model this situation as depicted in Figure 10 via shared transitions acquire1 and release1 used by the first nurse and acquire2 and release2 used by the second one. It takes at least *minReady* and at most *maxReady* time units to prepare the room for another patient.

Monitors. We use different types of monitors (small nets attached to the workflow) in order to observe executions of events and their temporal dependencies. Figure 11(a) shows how the execution of the event checkID and beginInfusionOf-BloodProduce can be registered by adding a component that will via shared transitions add a token to the place IDchecked resp. infusionStarted each time

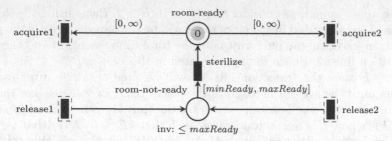

Fig. 10. Sharing of a resource (transfusion room example)

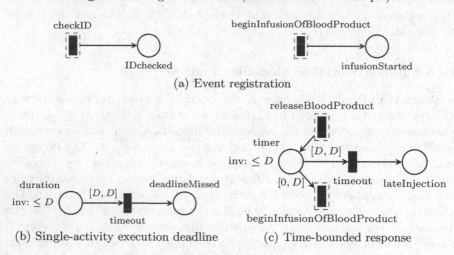

(a) Event registration

(b) Single-activity execution deadline   (c) Time-bounded response

Fig. 11. Monitors

the corresponding event is executed. Regarding temporal dependencies, observe that the nets for different Little-JIL primitives have a place (or several places) called duration. The duration place is marked by a token during the initialization of the activity and hence the age of the token represents the current execution time of the activity. We can add a monitor to such a duration place in order to check for the violation of the execution deadline D. The monitor is depicted in Figure 11(b) and it is clear that once the execution deadline D is reached, we are forced to mark the place deadlineMissed. Another type of monitor is given in Figure 11(c) where we can measure the response time between the events releaseBloodProduct and beginInfusionOfBloodProduct. Whenever the event releaseBloodProduct is not within D time units followed by the beginning of the transfusion, the place lateInjection gets marked.

4   Verification of the Blood Transfusion Case Study

Following the general algorithm presented in Section 3, we translated the blood transfusion case study described via Little-JIL diagrams into a component timed-arc Petri net and set up monitors for checking the crucial timing aspects of the workflow. The full set of Little-JIL diagrams and the manually created CTAPN models are available at the URL http://www.tapaal.net in the download section. For example, for the single-patient model, the composed net consists of 140 places, 98 transitions and 243 arcs.

We used the model checker TAPAAL [9] for the actual editing and verification of the CTAPN model. The tool offers a user-friendly GUI with the support for a fully automatic verification of a subset of TCTL that includes the temporal operators EF φ (a marking satisfying the proposition φ is reachable), AG φ (the proposition φ is satisfied in any reachable marking), EG φ (there is a maximal computation invariantly satisfying φ) and AF φ (on every maximal computation φ eventually holds). The formula φ consists of a boolean combination of atomic propositions of the form $P \le n$ and $P \ge n$ where P is a place and n is nonnegative integer, expressing the requirement that the number of tokens present in the place P is at most, resp. at least n.

We shall now present a selection of the verified queries for the blood transfusion case study; a full list of the queries is available within the TAPAAL model. Here workflow_END is the output place of the main workflow net and the other places are given in Figure 11. The place called duration corresponds to the overall duration of the whole workflow.

1. AG (infusionStarted=0 or IDchecked>=1) — ID is always checked at least once before the transfusion starts.
2. EF (workflow_END=1 and deadlineMissed=0) — The workflow can terminate within the deadline D (shortest execution time).
3. AG (workflow_END=1 or deadlineMissed=0) — In any scenario the workflow terminates within the deadline D (longest execution time).
4. AG lateInjection=0 — Late injection never happens (the time from picking up the blood product until the transfusion starts is not more that D time units; if $D = 30$ then this is exactly the B.9 property from the benchmark).
5. AF workflow_END=1 — Any maximal execution eventually reaches a marking where the whole workflow terminates (dynamical soundness).

Dynamical soundness implies that there are e.g. no deadlocks, no missing exception handlers and no improper use of the iteration activity. The temporal operator AF is a liveness operator and its verification is in general more demanding than the reachability and safety properties. We were able to positively verify this property for the whole workflow net in less than 10 second on a standard laptop; the other queries were positively verified in less than 1 second.[3] By varying the deadline D (declared as a constant in the net) we found out that the shortest execution time is 6 minutes (if patient disagrees with the transfusion), the longest execution time is 153 minutes and the longest time from picking up the blood product until its injection is 22 minutes (and hence the 30 minute expiration time imposed by B.9 property is met). Among the other properties

---

[3] All experiments were carried out by the native TAPAAL engines without using translations to UPPAAL timed automata that are also available in the tool.

we verified, we can e.g. mention that the shortest time of a successful transfusion is 118 minutes and we also successfully verified the property B.11 of the benchmark (patient is monitored during the transfusion every 15 minutes).

For two patients that share the same transfusion room, we confirmed in less than 40 seconds its dynamical soundness and verified that the longest execution time is 286 minutes. However, we found out that the B.9 property is broken. The tool provided an error trace showing a concrete execution of the workflow where the time from picking up the blood product until its injection exceeded 30 minutes. By examining the trace, we could easily find the reason: the pre-infusion activities allow in parallel to book the transfusion room and pick up the blood from the blood bank; as we might have to wait for the release of the transfusion room and its sterilization, the blood product can expire. This hints at the fact that, for more patients, these two activities have to be ordered sequentially.

A detailed comparison of the explicit state-space (discrete) verification methods and the DBM-based ones is beyond the scope of this paper but on the blood transfusion case study we can report that for the reachability properties the DBM-based methods were faster due to the higher constant sizes, whereas for liveness properties (dynamic soundness) the explicit methods were in this case considerably faster. A detailed comparison of the different verification methods is available in [3].

5   Conclusion

We have presented a general translation of medical healthcare workflows described in Little-JIL into component timed-arc Petri nets. As for any other workflow language, Little-JIL semantics can be conveniently given as a workflow Petri net via different constructions already described in the literature or via a direct translation into finite-state machines. The main contribution of our work is that we systematically model the *real-time aspects* of Little-JIL workflows and this allows us to use the tool TAPAAL for automatic verification of not only functional but also non-functional requirements as demonstrated on the blood transfusion case study.

The translation of the blood transfusion case study was performed manually but we are currently working on an automated tool for importing Little-JIL diagrams directly into TAPAAL. Another future research will focus on extending the property specification language and exploring how the technique will handle even larger case studies, including the possibility of direct code generation for automatic workflow coordination. On a different note, integrating human-specific aspects and ethical issues including security policies (like e.g. in OrBac [2]) into our approach is another challenge for the future work.

Acknowledgements. The work is partly supported by the projects GAVES, SAFEHR and EVGUI funded by the Macau Science and Technology Development Fund, and by MT-LAB, VKR Centre of Excellence. We thank to the anonymous reviewers for their detailed comments and suggestions.

References

1. Blood transfusion medical benchmark, `https://collab.cs.umass.edu/groups/laser_library/wiki/daf17/Blood_Transfusion_Medical_Benchmark.html`
2. Abou El Kalam, A., Baida, R.E., Balbiani, P., Benferhat, S., Cuppens, F., Deswarte, Y., Miège, A., Saurel, C., Trouessin, G.: Organization based access control. In: Policy 2003 (June 2003)
3. Andersen, M., Gatten Larsen, H., Srba, J., Grund Sørensen, M., Haahr Taankvist, J.: Verification of liveness properties on closed timed-arc petri nets. In: Kučera, A., Henzinger, T.A., Nešetřil, J., Vojnar, T., Antoš, D. (eds.) MEMICS 2012. LNCS, vol. 7721, pp. 69–81. Springer, Heidelberg (2013)
4. Bertolini, C., Schäf, M., Stolz, V.: Towards a Formal Integrated Model of Collaborative Healthcare Workflows. In: Liu, Z., Wassyng, A. (eds.) FHIES 2011. LNCS, vol. 7151, pp. 57–74. Springer, Heidelberg (2012)
5. Bolognesi, T., Lucidi, F., Trigila, S.: From timed Petri nets to timed LOTOS. In: 10th International Symposium on Protocol Specification, Testing and Verification, pp. 1–14. North-Holland, Amsterdam (1990)
6. Chen, B., Avrunin, G.S., Henneman, E.A., Clarke, L.A., Osterweil, L.J., Henneman, P.L.: Analyzing Medical Processes. In: ICSE 2008, pp. 623–632. ACM, New York (2008)
7. Chen, Z., Liu, Z., Ravn, A.P., Stolz, V., Zhan, N.: Refinement and verification in component-based model-driven design. Sci. Comp. Program. 74(4), 168–196 (2009)
8. Christov, S., Avrunin, G., Clarke, A., Osterweil, L., Henneman, E.: A benchmark for evaluating software engineering techniques for improving medical processes. In: Proceedings of the 2010 ICSE Workshop on Software Engineering in Health Care, SEHC 2010, pp. 50–56. ACM, New York (2010)
9. David, A., Jacobsen, L., Jacobsen, M., Jørgensen, K.Y., Møller, M.H., Srba, J.: TAPAAL 2.0: Integrated development environment for timed-arc Petri nets. In: Flanagan, C., König, B. (eds.) TACAS 2012. LNCS, vol. 7214, pp. 492–497. Springer, Heidelberg (2012)
10. del Foyo, P.M.G., Silva, J.R.: Using time Petri nets for modelling and verification of timed constrained workflow systems. In: ABCM Symposium Series in Mechatronics, vol. 3, pp. 471–478. ABCM (2008)
11. Grando, M.A., Glasspool, D.W., Fox, J.: Petri Nets as a Formalism for Comparing Expressiveness of Workflow-Based Clinical Guideline Languages. In: Ardagna, D., Mecella, M., Yang, J. (eds.) BPM 2008 Workshops. LNBIP, vol. 17, pp. 348–360. Springer, Heidelberg (2009)
12. Hanisch, H.-M.: Analysis of place/transition nets with timed-arcs and its application to batch process control. In: Ajmone Marsan, M. (ed.) ICATPN 1993. LNCS, vol. 691, pp. 282–299. Springer, Heidelberg (1993)
13. Jacobsen, L., Jacobsen, M., Møller, M.H., Srba, J.: Verification of timed-arc Petri nets. In: Černá, I., Gyimóthy, T., Hromkovič, J., Jefferey, K., Královič, R., Vukolić, M., Wolf, S. (eds.) SOFSEM 2011. LNCS, vol. 6543, pp. 46–72. Springer, Heidelberg (2011)
14. Jensen, K.: Coloured Petri Nets: Basic concepts, analysis methods and practical use. Springer, Berlin (1996)
15. Ke, W., Li, X., Liu, Z., Stolz, V.: rCOS: a formal model-driven engineering method for component-based software. Frontiers of Computer Science in China 6(1), 17–39 (2012)

16. Lamport, L.: Real-time model checking is really simple. In: Borrione, D., Paul, W. (eds.) CHARME 2005. LNCS, vol. 3725, pp. 162–175. Springer, Heidelberg (2005)
17. Ling, S., Schmidt, H.: Time Petri nets for workflow modelling and analysis. In: IEEE International Conference on Systems, Man and, Cybernetics, vol. 4, pp. 3039–3044. IEEE (2000)
18. MacCaull, W., Rabbi, F.: NOVA Workflow: A Workflow Management Tool Targeting Health Services Delivery. In: Liu, Z., Wassyng, A. (eds.) FHIES 2011. LNCS, vol. 7151, pp. 75–92. Springer, Heidelberg (2012)
19. Mashiyat, A.S., Rabbi, F., Wang, H., MacCaull, W.: An automated translator for model checking time constrained workflow systems. In: Kowalewski, S., Roveri, M. (eds.) FMICS 2010. LNCS, vol. 6371, pp. 99–114. Springer, Heidelberg (2010)
20. Merlin, P., Faber, D.: Recoverability of communication protocols: Implications of a theoretical study. IEEE Trans. on Communications 24(9), 1036–1043 (1976)
21. Miller, K., MacCaull, W.: Model checking timed properties of healthcare processes. Journal of Software Maintenance and Evolution: Research and Practice 23(4), 245–260 (2011)
22. OMG. UML extensions for workflow process definition - request for proposal. OMG-document bom/2000-12-11 (December 2000)
23. Rabbi, F., Mashiyat, A.S., MacCaull, W.: Model checking workflow monitors and its application to a pain management process. In: Liu, Z., Wassyng, A. (eds.) FHIES 2011. LNCS, vol. 7151, pp. 111–128. Springer, Heidelberg (2012)
24. Salimifard, K., Wright, M.: Petri net-based modelling of workflow systems: An overview. European Journal of Operational Research 134(3), 664–676 (2001)
25. van der Aalst, W.: The application of Petri nets to workflow management. The Journal of Circuits, Systems and Computers 8(1), 21–66 (1998)
26. van der Aalst, W., van Hee, K.: Workflow Management: Models, Methods, and Systems. MIT Press (2002)
27. van der Aalst, W., Weske, M., Wirtz, G.: Advanced topics in workflow management: Issues, requirements, and solutions. Journal of Integrated and Process Science 7(3), 49–77 (2003)
28. WFMC. Workflow management coalition terminology and glossary (WFMC-TC-1011). Technical report, Workflow Management Coalition, Brussels (1996)
29. Wise, A.: Little-JIL 1.5 language report (UM-CS-2006-51). Technical report, University of Massachusetts, Amherst, MA (2006)

Enhancing Product Line Development by Safety Requirements and Verification

Michaela Huhn and Sara Bessling

Department of Informatics, Clausthal University of Technology
Clausthal-Zellerfeld, Germany
{Michaela.Huhn,Sara.Bessling}@tu-clausthal.de

Abstract. In product lines of safety-critical medical devices, the safety requirements vary in the same lines as the products. We propose a uniform integration of safety requirements into a model-driven feature-oriented design methodology of product lines. We extend the SCADE development framework by a transformational approach to product line design: both the design modifications *and* the adaptation of safety requirements constitute a feature at a certain development phase. Thus both are described in terms of a model graph transformation. Then design models and the safety constraints associated to a product result from a sequence of feature-specific model transformations applied on a base model. This builds the basis for systematic and traceable product line verification and safety assurance. We evaluate our approach on a product line of cardiac pacemakers.

Keywords: Safety analysis, model-driven development, product lines.

1 Introduction

Software product line development addresses the engineering of families of similar products by means of systematically sharing development artifacts. In case of dependable products, safety requirements need to be specified and verified to hold for each product. Currently, the use of formal approaches to dependable systems product lines is hampered by (1) rather restrictive formal product building mechanisms and (2) a lack of support for the specification and verification of *product-specific* safety constraints that goes along with the design methodology. Both issues limit applicability of formal approaches to dependable systems product lines.

Feature models are a popular mean to specify variability in product lines at the problem space level at which the various stakeholders contribute with their requirements [20]. Feature models are often modeled as trees expressing a hierarchical decomposition of the products commonalities and differences along user-tangible product characteristics. A product of the product line is then described as an admissible combination of features.

In constructive development phases, the variability specification has to be linked to the artifacts of the solution space. In a model-driven approach to the development of software product lines, the design for variability and the composition of features forming a product have to be framed at the level of architectural and behavioral design models. As theoretically elaborated by Azanza et al. in [3], product generation can be

J. Weber and I. Perseil (Eds.): FHIES 2012, LNCS 7789, pp. 37–54, 2013.
© Springer-Verlag Berlin Heidelberg 2013

understood as a sequence of *endogenous* model transformations describing how a base model is transformed step-by-step into a specific product model. A transformation step corresponds to the modifications needed to realize a particular feature or feature group. It is formulated in terms of *model deltas* or *fragments* to be replaced. The transformation source (the base model) and the target (the product) conforms to the same metamodel, i.e. belong to the same viewpoint in the development process. Due to the flexibility of possible model transformations such transformational approaches support a broad variety of feature-specific adaptations [9,10,3] which is in contrast to other approaches using a single feature composition operator (see [2] for an overview). The Common Variability Language (CVL) by Haugen et al. [10] provides a tool that implements the transformational approach for the development of product lines based on EMF models.

One issue that has been addressed in the literature on dependable systems product lines is the verification of safety requirements common to *all* products of a product line as elaborated e.g. by [8,19], or [22] for a pacemaker product line. However, if features are considered a first class concept in product line development, their impact on the safety requirements to hold for its products is evident [15,5]. Thus, we propose to uniformly extend model transformations for variability design by the specification of feature-specific safety requirements. This means to consequently apply the principle of *reasoning along a system's major structuring concepts* for product lines also on the specification of safety requirements and their verification as it is done by architectural decomposition in traditional system design. Hence, when generating a product according to its selected features, the product design model *and* its safety requirements are created simultaneously. We demonstrate our approach within the SCADE development framework for the phases of architectural and functional design. We employ CVL to implement the model graph transformations for product generation. The case study on a product line for cardiac pacemakers shows that a transformational approach to product generation can deal with the different kinds of modifications needed for different features. Moreover, the systematic feature-specific fine-grained treatment seems to increase the portion of functionality covered by safety requirements.

The rest of the paper is structured as follows: Sec. 2 introduces SCADE and CVL which we use as the technical frameworks. In Sec. 3 we introduce the modeling of variability for architectural design models and model transformations to be applied on a base model. Moreover, we show that safety requirements can be handled analogously. Sec. 4 is dedicated to the case study of a pacemaker product line. Sec. 5 concludes.

2   Basics

2.1   Dependable System Modeling Using SCADE

The acronym SCADE stands for Safety-Critical Application Development Environment. The main objectives of the SCADE Suite are (1) to support systematic, model-based development of correct software based on formal methods and (2) to cover the whole development process [7]. The language *Scade* underlying the tool is data-flow oriented. Its formal semantics is based on a synchronous model of computation.

SCADE Suite is an integrated development environment that covers many development activities of a typical process for safety-critical software: modeling, formal verification using the SAT-based SCADE Design Verifier [1], certified automatic code generation producing readable and traceable C-code, requirements tracing down to model elements and code, simulation and testing on the code level and coverage metrics for the test cases with the Model Test Coverage module. The new version 6.3 of SCADE Suite integrates the SCADE System Designer that allows specifying the systems architecture by means of SysML block diagrams. The model entities of the System Designer project, i.e. blocks and connectors, are transformed into SCADE blocks and corresponding connections automatically.

Here we use SCADE System Designer to model the *structural* part of the design models and safety requirements, and SCADE Suite for the *behavioral* design and requirements modeling.

2.2 Variability Modeling Using CVL

The Common Variability Language (CVL) [10] facilitates the model driven development of product lines. CVL supports the specification of product variabilities upon a domain specific modeling language (DSL) defined by means of the Meta Object Facility (MOF). CVL separates the user-centric specification of variability, the *Feature Specification Layer* (FSL) from the developer-centric variability modeling, the *Product Realization Layer* (PRL). The PRL strictly follows a transformational approach.

At the Feature Specification Layer, CVL offers concepts that capture the usual hierarchical decomposition operators like *AND, OR, XOR, Mandatory* and *Optional* Features and *Cardinalities* known from many feature diagram notations (see [20] for an overview). The PRL associates local model graph transformations to the features describing how an individual feature is to be implemented in terms of *value, reference and fragment substitutions* applied on a *base model*. In general, a graph-based model transformation facilitates fine-grained feature-specific substitutions since a graph-based model transformation consists of an application context, i.e. a fragment to be removed from the model - called *the left hand side* of transformation - and the application condition *App*, and the fragment to be put in instead - called *the right hand side* of the transformation. A specific product is specified in the *Resolution Model* by selecting the features defining the product. The corresponding model transformation is yield by executing the substitutions associated with the selected features on the domain-specific base model in a predefined order.

We employ CVL for feature modeling of a pacemaker product line and the transformational approach for the product line design and the representation of feature-specific safety requirements.

2.3 Related Work

Numerous approaches deal with variability management in the design space by associating model (or code) fragments to product features. In order to build a product, a base model is adapted as prescribed by the model fragments. Thereby "adaptation" may be interpreted as *adding* the fragments to a minimal model, or as *subtracting* fragments not needed from a 150 % model, or other kinds of *composition*, see [2,3] for detailed surveys. Transformational approaches like e.g. [10,3] describe the model adaptations corresponding to each feature in terms of model transformations. Graph transformational approaches support feature-specific modifications that may refer to a specific application context. However, these approaches focus on structural design models, but do not consider behavioral safety requirements and their verification.

Liu et al. [16,15] work on safety analysis and verification techniques dedicated for product lines. Liu et al. define a flexible, *sequential* composition on transition systems which represent the base model's or a feature's behavior. They propose a compatible, automated decomposition of temporal formulae for model checking: At the *variation points*, the states at which the system "traverses" from the behavior of feature A to that of feature B, proof obligations are calculated for the transition system belonging to the features entered next. As we do, Liu et al. consider a product line of pacemakers as a case study. Compared to our synchronous product, the sequential composition is less flexible as it assumes that exactly one feature is active at any moment. The explicit reference to features in the safety requirements is another difference to our approach: We handle the generation of a design model and the related safety requirements uniformly, hence the safety requirements are specific for a selected feature combination without explicitly referring to the resulting product.

Classen et al. [6,5] propose *feature transition systems* as a formal low-level behavioral model that captures all products of a product line by labelling each transition with a Boolean expression describing for which features this transition may be selected. The approach focusses on verification and is independent from the design methodology.

Several approaches are on target for formal verification of cardiac pacemakers: Tuan, Zheng, and Tho [22] give high-level models of several pacemakers in terms of CSP. They verify five safety properties common to most of them like deadlock freedom, or upper and lower rate limits. Jiang et al. [14] model a DDD pacemaker with two specific anti-PMT algorithms in detail. They work with timed automata using UPPAAL in order to verify that the pacemaker reacts correctly in specific situations of tachycardia. A detailed Event-B modeling of pacemakers can be found in [17]. Refinement is applied to incrementally add functional and timing properties to the abstract system-level specification. The properties to be verified address the system architecture, action-reaction and the timing behavior of several pacemaker variants. Jee et al. [13,12] use UPPAAL in order to formally develop and verify the software control of pacemakers. Therefore they have extended UPPAAL by a synthesis to C-Code. In [12], a product-centric assurance case for the pacemakers is investigated which requires a thoughtful combination of methods and results from safety analysis, design and verification. Liu et al. [15] and Jee et al. [12] use other formalisms than we do, but the intended seamless integration of safety analysis, development, and verification is similar to our approach.

3   Adding Variability to Dependable System Development

3.1   The Base Model and Models Deltas

We build our product line models upon an architectural component model represented in terms of SysML blocks. Due to the SysML Specification [18], blocks are well-suited to "define a collection of features to describe a system". We restrict ourselves to a subset of SysML Block Definition Diagrams (bdd) and Internal Block Diagrams (ibd) as

they are supported by SCADE System Designer. A Block Definition Diagram describes
the architectural decomposition into *blocks* representing (sub)systems to be realized in
software or hardware.

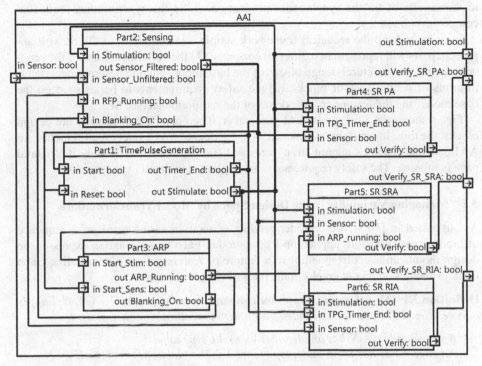

Fig. 1. The ibd for the AAI pacemaker

The Internal Block Diagrams model the *parts*[1] within a block and their interfaces by
typed *ports* with a direction *in* or *out*. Behavior is allocated to parts using SCADE in
the *functional design* phase. We denote the behavioral model associated with a structural part A, its SCADE node, by *A*. *Connectors* represent the communication either
between internal parts of blocks by linking ports or the in/output of a composite block
by a connection to an external port. Connectors are restricted to compatible interfaces,
i.e. ports with compatible types and matching direction. The block behavior is modeled in SCADE (see Fig. 7 for illustration). Thus, the behavior of a block A is defined
as the *synchronous product*, denoted Π, of all its sub-blocks at which each connector
from bdd B.outp1 to C.inp2 is interpreted as an additional equation that relates
the output variable *outp*1 of the behavior associated with B with the input *inp*2 of C's
associated block, i.e. *B.outp*1 = *C.inp*2. Connectors to the external ports of a block are
handled accordingly. Thus, the behavioral model specified in an ibd A is syntactically
given as

$$A = \prod\nolimits_{B\ partof\ A} B \oplus Connect\_EqA \qquad (1)$$

---

[1] As sub-blocks are called in SysML.

where *Connect_EqA* denotes the set of equations induced by the connectors of A and ⊕ the syntactic addition of these equations to the syntactic behavior representations of the parts of A. We note that in case blocks are unconnected, the synchronous product semantically yields parallel composition, in case all outports of a part B1 are connected to the inports of B2 the synchronous product results in the synchronous, sequential composition B1;B2.

In order to keep the technical framework simple and compliant to the SCADE approach, parts will represent two different concepts: (1) the building entities of the product line, i.e. the structural design blocks of the base model and the design model deltas in terms of feature-specific blocks, (2) the safety requirements to be satisfied on the base model and the feature-specific deltas of the requirements (see Sec. 3.3).

Fig. 1 shows the ibd for an AAI pacemaker: The upper left three parts are design blocks, the three lower right ones named "SR..." denote AAI's safety requirements. An AAI pacemaker senses natural atrial paces and stimulates the atrium only if a natural pace is missing. The safety requirements are explained in detail in chapter 4.4.

3.2 Managing Variability in the Design Space by Model Transformations

As suggested in [10,3], we consider product generation as the result of a sequence of model transformations applied on a base model. Each transformation expresses the design modifications corresponding to a feature or feature group. We formalize graph transformations on model graphs in the lines of [23] as follows:

Definition 3.1 (Model graph, graph morphism). *A model graph $G = \langle N, E, Lab \rangle$ is a finite, directed, typed and attributed graph with the following constraints.*

- *A graph node $n \in N$ has an identifier* Id, *and a type label* T_n.
- *An edge $e \in E$ has an* Id *and a type label* T_e. *The functions $src, tgt : E \to N$ give its source and target, resp.*
- *Both nodes and edges may be associated with attributes (represented e.g. as special graph nodes), with an* Id *identifier, a type label* T_a *and a data value (default).*
- *Lab denotes the labeling of nodes and edges.*

Let G, H be two model graphs. In the following we denote the obvious extension of a set-theoretic operation op to graphs by op^g : e.g. the intersection of graph G and H is defined as $\langle N_G \cap N_H, E_G \cap E_H, Lab\lceil_{N_G \cap N_H, E_G \cap E_H} \rangle$ and denoted $G \cap^g H$.

A graph morphism $f : G \to^g H$ is a structure-preserving (total) function, i.e $src_H \circ f\lceil_{E_G} = f\lceil_{N_G} \circ src_G, tgt_H \circ f\lceil_{E_G} = f\lceil_{N_G} \circ tgt_G$, and Lab_H extends $f \circ Lab_G$.

EMF models and hence the SysML diagrams we use for architectural modeling can be canonically mapped onto model graphs as explained in [23]: Instances of EMF entities are mapped to graph nodes with the same name and type. Links between the EMF model entities are usually non-directed, thus they are mapped on two graph edges between the corresponding nodes. Attributes are mapped one-to-one.

Definition 3.2 (Transformation rule). *A graph transformation rule is a tuple $r = \langle L, R, App \rangle$ consisting of a left hand side (LHS) graph L, a right hand side (RHS) graph R, and the application constraint App. The intersection of L and R, i.e. the graph $I = L \cap^g R$ is called the* interface *of the rule r.*

The idea of a transformation rule $r = \langle L, R, App \rangle$ is to replace an occurrence of the LHS L in G by the RHS R provided the application constraint App is satisfied on G. Thereby the nodes and edges from $L \setminus^g R$ will be deleted, those from $R \setminus^g L$ will be added and the interface I builds the "glue" which is called *boundary declaration* in CVL [10]. We say r is *applicable* to the host graph G if there exists a graph morphism called *match* $m : L \to^g G$, such that

- m is an injective graph morphism,
- For all $e \in E_G$, $src(e) \in m(N_L \setminus N_R)$ or $tgt(e) \in m(N_L \setminus N_R)$ implies $e \in m(E_L \setminus E_R)$ (no dangling edges)
- The predicate App evaluates to $\mathtt{true}$ on G.

Let $G = \langle N, E, Lab \rangle$ be a model graph and $r = \langle L, R, App \rangle$ be a transformation rule applicable on G and m a match for the LHS L on G.

Definition 3.3 (Application of a transformation rule). *The application of r on G at the match m is defined using an extension of m to a morphism $m' : L \cup^g R \to^g H$ such that H extends G and all nodes and edges from $R \setminus^g L$ are mapped by m' to fresh and distinct elements of $H \setminus^g G$ and the resulting* target *graph H is defined by*

$$H = (G \setminus^g m(L)) \cup^g m'(R).$$

To illustrate the transformations assigned to features we consider the feature *Dual_P* in *Chambers paced* (see Fig. 4). *Dual_P* specifies the feature of generating artificial pulses for both heart chambers. Since we have chosen a single chamber pacemaker, namely $\mathtt{AAI}$, as the base model, the design model transformation assigned to *Dual_P* adds a second pulse generation part to the base model as depicted in Fig. 2. The $\mathtt{AAI}$ $\mathtt{block}$ forms the graph interface; thus it occurs on the LHS and the RHS.

The entities to be added are represented as the RHS of the transformation, for simplicity we have omitted the association_start and _end attributes at the edges: a Boolean output $\mathtt{Stimulate}$ of the block is added. A new part $\mathtt{TPG}$, which abbreviates $\mathtt{TimePulseGeneration}$ (see Fig. 1), is added with the appropriate in- and outports $\mathtt{Start}$, $\mathtt{Reset}$, $\mathtt{Stimulate}$, and $\mathtt{Timer\_running}$. The internal outport $\mathtt{Stimulate}$ is linked to the corresponding outport of the pacemaker $\mathtt{Stimulate}$ via a connector which is remains unnamed in Fig. 2 and the $\mathtt{Timer\_running}$ outport is connected to the $\mathtt{Start}$ inport of $\mathtt{TPG}$ via another unnamed connector (please compare this to the part in Fig. 1). The edges denote links between associated model concepts like those between a part and its ports, etc.

If applied, the transformation rule results in a fresh $\mathtt{TimePulseGeneration}$ part with all ports and connections needed. In order to generate the parts of the ibds corresponding to the safety requirements associated with the *Dual_P* feature, the rule has to be extended accordingly which we leave out for brevity here.

We employ the CVL tool [10] to implement the model transformations for architectural design models specified in SCADE System Designer. CVL provides a mechanism to specify and execute so-called substitutions on domain-specific MOF-based models. A *substitution* consists of (1) the *placement fragment* which corresponds to the LHS of a transformation rule, (2) the *replacement fragment* representing the RHS, and (3) the *boundary declaration* that conceptually replaces the interface of the rule.

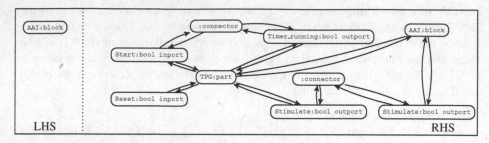

Fig. 2. Model transformation for the design part of the *Dual_P* feature

3.3 A Uniform Enhancement by Safety Requirements

In feature-oriented product line development, safety requirements on a product naturally relate to the functionality that is provided by its features. When looking on all products in a body, this relation sometimes is expressed by explicit references to features in the properties to be verified: e.g. by constraining a safety property by a predicate indicating the presence of a specific feature as done in [15] or in [5].

We uniformly extend the handling of variability in the design space to the specification of safety requirements and verification. Thus we employ the mechanism used for product generation, namely model transformation, to create the safety requirements that are specific for the selected features defining the product.

The conceptual precondition is that safety requirements constitute a proper viewpoint in the model driven development that is captured in a model. SCADE fulfills this precondition immediately: In SCADE, a safety requirement is expressed as an observer node which is syntactically the same as any design node. Semantically, an observer is an additional node which concurrently monitors the design and checks for safety violations. Thus, it is handled as yet another block in the synchronous product as defined in Eq. 1. However, one could argue that separate concepts, namely the architectural design and the safety requirements, should be expressed using different modeling concepts; for instance, the *SysML requirements and constraint* concepts (see [18] Chap. 16) could be used for safety requirements. To support separate modeling concepts, the modeling facilities for the base model and the model deltas as well as the model transformation would have to be extended by a "requirement" metamodel. We avoided this extension here, because a separated "requirement" metamodel raises technical complexity, but without any effect on the back-end, the SCADE Suite, which we use for functional design and verification.

We proceed methodically as follows: First we identify the safety requirements for the base model (see Fig. 1) which shall cover basic functionality common to all products of the product line as well as constraints that are specific for the features present in the base model. Then the adaptations of safety requirements associated with a feature are described as requirement deltas, i.e. the model transformation to be applied on the base models is extended to the safety requirements. Product generation, i.e. performing the sequence of model transformations then yields both, an architectural design model and observer nodes representing the product's safety requirements in terms of SysML block diagrams.

In our opinion, adding safety requirements per feature has two main advantages: First, the set of safety requirements $SafeReq_F$ specific for feature F are generated for each product at which the feature F is present. Thus, in case one of them is violated due to unwanted feature interaction with other features assigned to a specific product the violation will be discovered as soon as verification is performed. Second, software safety requirements are the outcome of software safety analysis. As safety analysis techniques like FTA (Fault Tree Analysis) or FMEA (Failure Mode and Effect Analysis) often follow architectural decomposition, a feature-specific procedure appears to be well-suited for feature-oriented product lines development.

3.4 Behavioral Models and Verification

Variability modeling by model transformations applies to the architectural design phase. The functional behavior is added for both the design models and the observer nodes representing the safety requirements in the *functional design* phase using SCADE.

The semantics of a compound SCADE model is formalized in terms of transition systems as described in [1]. Thus, the formal behavioral semantics $[\![A]\!]$ of an ibd A with the associated SCADE model A is given via Eq. 1 as

$$[\![A]\!] = [\![A]\!] = [\![\textstyle\prod_{B\,part of\,A} B \oplus Connect\_EqA]\!] = \langle S_A, I_A, \rightarrow_A \rangle \tag{2}$$

where S_A is the set of states built from the synchronous product of A's sub-blocks, $I_A \subseteq S_A$ is the set of initial states, and $\rightarrow_A \subseteq S_A \times S_A$ is the transition relation. Based on the transition system semantics, SCADE Design Verifier provides SAT-based model checking that seamlessly enables to verify reachability properties. When verification is applied on the behavioral design module A and any observer node $A.SR\_id$ we yield that either the safety property expressed by $A.SR\_id$ holds on all reachable states of $[\![A]\!]$ or a trace $s_1, s_2, \ldots s_n$ is generated from the model checker that witnesses a violation. Thus, as soon as the functional design is completed and the safety requirements are specified as observer nodes, the verification of all product-specific safety properties can be performed.

3.5 Implementation of the Graph Transformational Approach

The graph transformation as it is used here is an endogenous model graph transformation based on a relatively simple metamodel of SysML block diagrams. Thus, the application to product lines is straightforward from the theoretical viewpoint and from the methodological point of view we follow and refine the ideas from [3].

Technically, the handling of SCADE block diagrams raises little additional effort in CVL, as CVL already provides support for SysML model elements based on EMF. However, defining the substitutions is technically sophisticated as it requires a very detailed understanding of the SysML metamodel and the functioning of a CVL substitution on a SysML model instance. Both are presented implicitly only in CVL. Consequently, the ingredients of a substitution, the placement, the replacement and the boundary elements, are often defined incompletely or ambiguously which leads to manual redefinitions within the substitution that was generated by CVL. The substitution explicitly describes all modifications that have to be executed in order to generate the target model as an instance of the metamodel from the source model, including all attributes and relations of the model elements used. One may imagine that a manual reworking of this description becomes laborious.

4   Variability in a Pacemaker Product Line

4.1   The Pacemaker Product Line

Industrial pacemakers are categorized by an international code, the NASPE/BPEG Code [4]. Its definition enfolds five letters. The first three letters characterize the main functions of a pacemaker as the stimulation of the heart, the detection of natural heart pace and the response mode to detection. The letters indicate the heart chambers affected by stimulation or detection, resp., i.e. "A" denotes *atrial* stimulation, "V" a *ventricular* one, "D" is used for *dual* chamber pacing and "0" indicates *none*. For the response mode, "0" denotes *none*, "I" the *inhibited* mode in which a sensed natural pace inhibits artificial pacing and "T" the *triggered* mode in which a sensed natural pace triggers an immediate artificial pace. The response mode "D" combines the response modes inhibited and triggered: A natural atrial pace inhibits an artificial atrial pace. Moreover, an (artificial or natural) atrial pace triggers an artificial ventricular pace at the end of the so-called AV interval[2] (AVI), in case no natural ventricular pulse is sensed in between.

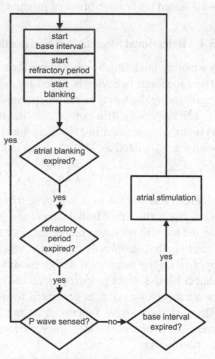

Fig. 3. Flowchart of the AAI pacemaker

An AAI pacemaker is a variant that stimulates the atrium, in case no atrial pace is detected. A base interval (BI), an atrial refractory period (ARP) and a blanking time are started at every cycle of an AAI pacemaker (as shown in Fig. 3). During the blanking time, which is an initial part of the refractory period, nothing is sensed at all; during the ARP natural paces are sensed but not considered in the pacemalder's decision for stimulation. After the end of the ARP the pacemaker awaits a natural pace until the end of the base interval. If and only if no natural pace is sensed until the BI expires the pacemaker will trigger an atrial stimulation. Then the BI starts anew.

In difference, a DDD pacemaker senses and stimulates both chambers. At the beginning of each cycle a BI for the atrium and a corresponding ARP start in combination with an AVI for the ventricle. The AVI and the ARP have the same length. During the AVI the pacemaker awaits a ventricular pace and if this does not occur until the end

---

[2] The AV interval is the maximum time between an atrial pace and a ventricular one.

of the AVI, a ventricular stimulation is triggered. After this a ventricular refractory period (VRP) starts, as well as a second atrial refractory period called PVARP. ARP and VRP except PVARP contain a blanking period. The pacemaker then awaits an atrial pace until the end of the BI. Furthermore a ventricular blanking period starts after each atrial event and after each ventricular event an atrial blanking period, preventing cross-sensing. The DDD pacemaker can detect a ventricular extra-systole (VES). A VES is a natural ventricular pace without a preceding atrial event and needs an exceptional treatment. This results in a special cycle in which only the base interval and the refractory periods except PVARP start anew. Furthermore, the DDD variant comes with a hysteresis functionality changing the length of the AV interval after an artificial pace. The final two letters of NASPE/BPEG Code describe additional features like a possible rate modulation or multisite stimulation of a heart chamber. For brevity, we will restrict the case study to a subset of the three mandatory functional groups mentioned so far. However, we consider an additional variant of the DDD pacemaker, called DDDR, that enables rate modulation of pacing. Moreover, the dual pacemakers implement a so-called *hysteresis* which adapts the AV interval depending on the kind of ventricular pace that has been sensed in the previous cycle. Some pacemakers offer functions to detect and react on sporadic atrial tachycardia, e.g. by showing a behavior similar to a Wenckebach anomaly. However, we do not consider such functionality here. Mode switches are ignored as well. All behavioral details and an informal specification of the safety requirements originate from an industrial specification by Boston Scientific [21].

We use the NASPE/BPEG Code to structure the features of pacemakers as shown in Fig. 4. The mandatory functionality for stimulation, sensing and the sensing response mode specify the feature groups on the first layer. At the second layer a single feature is selected from each group (XOR operator).

4.2 The Pacemaker's Base Model and Model Deltas

The AAI pacemaker builds our base model. Its `ibd` is depicted in Fig. 1. The main design part `TimePulseGeneration` decides for generating a pulse at the end of the *base interval* (BI). The `Sensing` part filters the signals from the sensor and signals detection of a natural pace to the other parts.

The `Atrial Refractory Period` (ARP) part realizes a deactivation of both stimulation and detection after a natural or artificial pulse. Neither a stimulation nor a sensing of the heart must occur within the refractory interval as both would be safety-critical: Sensing shortly after a pulse may lead to misinterpretation, pacing may cause life-threatening cardiac fibrillation. The other parts in the `ibd` of AAI represent the safety requirements for each feature and are explained in Section 4.4.

4.3 Model Transformations for Product Generation

At the product realization layer of CVL, variability is described in terms of transformations on the base model, notably, the AAI pacemaker. The simpler variant A00 stimulates the heart periodically at the end of the BI without sensing natural paces and without response mode, which is represented by the features *None* in the feature groups *Sensing* and *Sensing response*. The corresponding transformations remove the parts `Sensing`

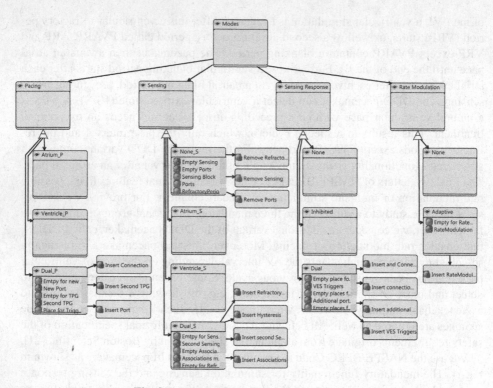

Fig. 4. Pacemaker feature diagram as CVL tree

and `ARP`, as well as the corresponding inputs for sensing, several connections and the inport "Reset" of the part `TimePulseGeneration`. The V00 pacemaker is generated with the same transformations for the feature groups *Chambers sensed* and *Sensing response* as the A00 pacemaker. In the feature group *Pacing* the feature "Ventricle" is chosen in which the only transformation is an adaptation of time intervals.

The third pacemaker product considered is the D00 pacemaker using the features "None" from the feature groups *Sensing* and *Sensing response*. The feature "Dual" in the feature group *Pacing* leads to a doubling of the `TimePulse Generation` as well as of the "Stimulation" output and connects both `TimePulse Generation` parts in order to synchronize the atrial and the ventricular pacing.

The VVI pacemaker is nearly identical to the AAI pacemaker. Configuration parameters are adopted only in order to build a VVI pacemaker from the AAI base model.

The DDD pacemaker design is derived from the AAI base model by essentially doubling all functions: Furthermore a new block named `VES` is introduced that handles extra-ordinary natural pulses of the ventricle. If a VES is sensed, the `VES` block triggers a reset of the atrial `TimePulseGeneration` and both `RefractoryPeriod` blocks. Moreover, a `Hysteresis` block and a block for the `PVARP` timer are added. The `PVARP` timer is started after an artificial or natural ventricular pace and serves as additional block for the atrial sensor lest no misinterpretation of ventricular signals may occur. For the DDDR pacemaker we assume that rate modulation is based on an activity sensor that measures the ventricular pressure using a piezoelectric crystal and can be incorporated into the pacing lead. The piezoelectric sensor yields a voltage that is used as an input by the `RateModulation` block for altering the base interval accordingly.

4.4 Variability of Safety Requirements

From the safety analysis we derive several safety requirements for the each variant. Each safety requirement can be assigned to a specific feature group. The safety requirements differ not only with respect to the functionality but we also have variations of the real-time constants they refer to.

- Safety requirements for *Pacing*
  - *At most one pace (PA/PV)* Within the base interval (BI) at most one atrial/ventricular artificial pace occurs[3].
  - *The AV synchrony is respected (PSyn)* An artificial ventricular pace is only triggered if the AV interval (AVI) is expired.
- Safety requirements for *Sensing* the chambers
  - *Refractory period (SA/SV)* During a refractory period of the atrium/ventricle neither a pace detection nor a stimulation occurs[4].
- Safety requirements for the *Response* on the sensing
  - *Strict artificial pacing (R0A/R0V)* During the BI, an artificial atrial/ventricular pace is triggered exactly once.
  - *The AV synchrony is respected (RSyn)* The period between the atrial and ventricular artificial pacing is exactly AVI.
  - *Natural pace inhibits artificial pace (RIA/RIV)* Iff no natural atrial/ventricular pace is detected within the admissible intervals of the BI, an artificial atrial/ventricular pace is triggered exactly once.
  - *AV synchrony and ventricular inhibition (RSynIV)* After an atrial pace a natural ventricular pace is awaited in the interval [0,AVI), in case the natural ventricular pace is missing, at time AVI an artificial ventricular pace is triggered.
  - *Response on an ventricular extra-systole (RVES)* If a natural ventricular pace occurs in the interval $[AVI + VRP, BI[$[5] then neither an artificial atrial pace nor an artificial ventricular pace is triggered from this occurrence t_0 on until time $t_0 + BI$.
  - *Rate Modulation (RM)* Although in the presence of Rate Modulation the actual BI is always within the limits defined by the Upper (URL) and the Lower Rate Limit (LRL).

The AAI pacemaker shall satisfy three safety requirements, namely PA, SA and RIA. These are generated as observer nodes as parts of the base model. The VVI pacemaker has the requirements PV, SV and RIV. These are identical to the ones from the AAI pacemaker, except that they refer to the ventricle timing instead of the atrium. The A00

---

[3] The two safety requirements refer to different outports.
[4] As the atrial and ventricular refractory periods differ, the time interval in the safety requirements have to be adapted accordingly, too.
[5] VRP is the time interval of the ventricular refractory period.

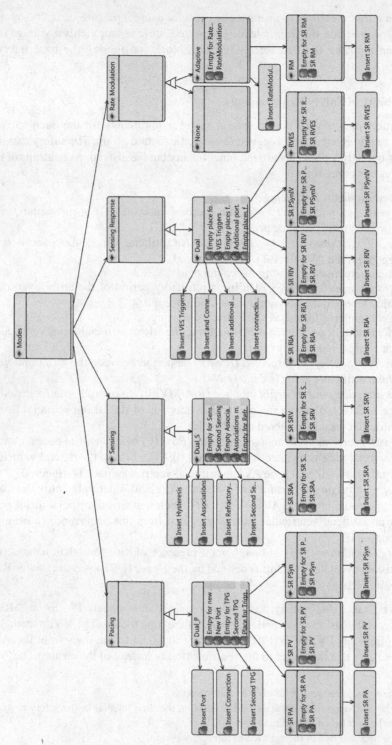

Fig. 5. Detail of CVL tree for DDD(R) pacemaker

pacemaker possesses only two safety constraints PA and R0A. They are derived from PA and RIA, respectively, by eliminating the parts for the natural pacing. The safety requirements of the V00 pacemaker are PV and R0V, respectively.

The D00 pacemaker stimulates atrium and ventricle. Therefore we need two safety requirements for each chamber and the strict synchronization between atrial and ventricular pacing. These are namely PA, PV, PSyn, R0A, R0V, and RSyn.

For the DDD pacemaker we duplicate the safety requirements of the AAI pacemaker to adapt to the dual sensing and pacing of the atrium and the ventricle. The RSynIV safety requirement guarantees atrial controlled ventricular pacing at the end of the AV interval. Furthermore, we add a safety requirement RVES for the VES feature. Fig. 5 gives an overview of the safety requirements belonging to the DDD features.

4.5 Behavioral Modeling in SCADE

When synchronizing the SysML models that result from the CVL transformation with SCADE Suite generates the corresponding (bare) operators (see Fig. 6).

For each pacemaker, a SCADE operator is created as well as inner operators for both kinds of blocks, the design and the observers. SysML connectors are mapped to connections representing the equa-

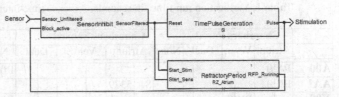

Fig. 6. SCADE diagram of the AAI pacemaker (design parts)

tions to implement the connector semantics as defined in Sec. 3.1, Eq. 1. This generation of SCADE operators is done automatically by the SCADE System Designer by importing the SysML model files per a special interface.

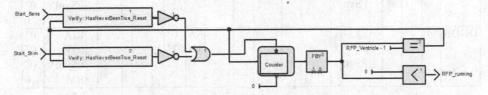

Fig. 7. SCADE operator of the design part `RefractoryPeriod`

Behavioral modeling is done in SCADE manually for the base model and each model delta, i.e. each design operator and each observer node expressing a safety constraint is modeled as prescribed in the functional specification. For instance, Fig. 7 shows the SCADE node for the `RefractoryPeriod`. The counter is triggered by an input and runs until it reaches the constant *RFP_Ventricle*. Then a reset is triggered.

Fig. 8 shows the SCADE operator which corresponds to the safety requirement SR `RefractoryPeriod` denoted SRA and SRV, resp., in Sec. 4.4. The output *Proof* switches to false if the refractory period is active and at the same time a natural pace is sensed or a stimulation occurs.

4.6   Verification of Products

Table 1 shows the verification results. The safety requirements are structured along the feature groups. An empty field indi-

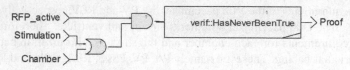

Fig. 8. Safety requirement SR_RefractoryPeriod as SCADE operator

cates that there is no safety requirement specific to that feature on this product. The figures indicate the run-times of a successful proof by SCADE Design Verifier executed on a Intel Core 2 Duo P9700 2,80 GHz. Most constraints - except those on refractory periods - could be verified nearly instantaneously. In order to prove some of the more involved safety requirements of the DDD pacemaker we rescaled the timing constants by a factor 1:10, because only then we were able to achieve verification results in a reasonable time.

Table 1. Verification run-times in seconds, * means time intervals divided by 10

	Chambers Paced						Chambers Sensed								Sensing Response					
	Atrium		Ventr.		Dual		None	Atrium		Ventr.		Dual		None		Inhibit		Dual	
A00	PA	0												R0A	0				
AAI	PA	0						SA	5379							RIA	0		
V00			PV	0										R0V	0				
VVI			PV	0						SV	4391					RIV	0		
D00					PA	0								R0A	0				
					PV	0								R0V	0				
					PSyn	0								RSyn	0				
DDD					PA	0						SA	0*					RIA	3*
					PV	0						SV	4*					RIV	10*
					PSyn	0												PSynIV	0*
																	RVES	0
DDDR					PA	1						SA	0*					RIA	0*
					PV	1						SV	22*					RIV	0*
					PSyn	1												PSynIV	0*
																	RM	0

The most evident observation from the case study is that reuse of submodels as well as feature-specific singularities can be found in the design models as well as in the safety requirements: The basic pacing constraints PA and PV, for its ventricular counterpart resp., apply to all products, whereas only the DDD pacemaker needs to deal with the RVES requirement.

Next, we compare the verification results to our previous work on the verification of monolithic data-flow-oriented pacemaker models [11]. In [11], we derived the pacemaker variants more informally from each other. But we could *not* produce verification results for most constraints by just using SCADE Design Verifier due to complexity problems. Only when applying time abstraction by transferring the verification problem to UPPAAL, we could prove the pacemakers correct. Thus the product line approach apparently has a positive impact on verification: The strict structuring of both design and observer models in the base model and the fragments seems to fit well to SCADE Design Verifier's built-in heuristics for speeding up verification.

Another observation is that the feature-specific modeling of safety deltas leads to more detailed safety requirements. Hence, the portion of the pacemaker's behavior that is covered by safety constraints increases compared to a top level specification of safety constraints on all products in a body.

5 Conclusion

We presented a transformational model-based approach to product line design for safety-critical systems that uniformly handles design models *and* safety requirements. We used graph transformations to describe the modifications needed to adapt a base design model *and* its safety requirements according to a feature. We demonstrated the approach within the SCADE framework for the modeling and verification of dependable medical device software and employed CVL for transformational product generation.

Product line development is commonly used in the medical device domain in order to adapt the products to the characteristic requirements needed for individual patients or variants of a disease. SCADE Suite provides certified code generation for dependable systems according to several safety standards and, moreover, formal verification by STA-based model checking. Thus our approach is supported by a tool offering seamless model-based development and is approved in practice. For the pacemaker case study, we could successfully prove all safety requirements to hold on the pacemaker variants which is due to the limited functionality of pacemaker software. We believe that our promising results on verification, which are in contrast to other domains at which verification heavily suffers from complexity problems, transfers to a number of other medical devices which are of restricted complexity as well.

Our next step is to introduce concepts for failure modeling and a feature-oriented safety analysis methodology.

References

1. Abdulla, P.A., Deneux, J., Stålmarck, G., Ågren, H., Åkerlund, O.: Designing safe, reliable systems using Scade. In: Margaria, T., Steffen, B. (eds.) ISoLA 2004. LNCS, vol. 4313, pp. 115–129. Springer, Heidelberg (2006)
2. Apel, S., Kästner, C.: An overview of feature-oriented software development. Journal of Object Technology 8(5), 49–84 (2009)
3. Azanza, M., Batory, D., Díaz, O., Trujillo, S.: Domain-specific composition of model deltas. In: Tratt, L., Gogolla, M. (eds.) ICMT 2010. LNCS, vol. 6142, pp. 16–30. Springer, Heidelberg (2010)
4. Bernstein, Daubert, Fletcher, Hayes, Lüderitz, Reynolds, Schoenfeld, Sutton: The revised NASPE/BPEG generic code for antibradycardia, adaptive-rate, and multisite pacing. Journal of Pacing and Clinical Electrophysiology 25, 260–264 (2002)
5. Classen, A., Heymans, P., Schobbens, P.Y., Legay, A.: Symbolic model checking of software product lines. In: Intern. Conf. on Software Engineering (ICSE), pp. 321–330 (2011)

6. Classen, A., Heymans, P., Schobbens, P.Y., Legay, A., Raskin, J.F.: Model checking lots of systems: efficient verification of temporal properties in software product lines. In: Intern. Conf. on Software Engineering (ICSE), pp. 335–344 (2010)
7. Esterel Technologies: SCADE Suite KCG 6.1: Safety case report of KCG 6.1.2 (July 2009)
8. Fischbein, D., Uchitel, S., Brabermann, V.: A foundation for behavioural conformance in software product line architectures. In: ISSTA 2006 Workshop on Role of Software Architecture for Testing and Analysis (ROSATEA), pp. 39–48. ACM (2006)
9. Gray, J., Zhang, J., Lin, Y., Roychoudhury, S., Wu, H., Sudarsan, R., Gokhale, A., Neema, S., Shi, F., Bapty, T.: Model-driven program transformation of a large avionics framework. In: Karsai, G., Visser, E. (eds.) GPCE 2004. LNCS, vol. 3286, pp. 361–378. Springer, Heidelberg (2004)
10. Haugen, Møller-Pedersen, Oldevik, Olsen, Svendsen: Adding standardized variability to domain specific languages. In: Intern. Software Product Line Conference, pp. 139–148. IEEE Computer Society (2008)
11. Huhn, M., Bessling, S.: Towards certifiable software for medical devices: The pacemaker case study revisited. In: Intern. Workshop on Harnessing Theories for Tool Support in Software, pp. 8–14 (2011)
12. Jee, E., Lee, I., Sokolsky, O.: Assurance cases in model-driven development of the pacemaker software. In: Margaria, T., Steffen, B. (eds.) ISoLA 2010, Part II. LNCS, vol. 6416, pp. 343–356. Springer, Heidelberg (2010)
13. Jee, Wang, Kim, Lee, Sokolsky, Lee: A safety-assured development approach for real-time software. In: Proceedings of the 2010 IEEE 16th International Conference on Embedded and Real-Time Computing Systems and Applications, pp. 133–142. IEEE Computer Society, Washington, DC (2010), http://dx.doi.org/10.1109/RTCSA.2010.42
14. Jiang, Z., Pajic, M., Moarref, S., Alur, R., Mangharam, R.: Modeling and verification of a dual chamber implantable pacemaker. In: Flanagan, C., König, B. (eds.) TACAS 2012. LNCS, vol. 7214, pp. 188–203. Springer, Heidelberg (2012)
15. Liu, J., Basu, S., Lutz, R.R.: Compositional model checking of software product lines using variation point obligations. Autom. Softw. Eng. 18(1), 39–76 (2011)
16. Liu, J., Dehlinger, J., Lutz, R.R.: Safety analysis of software product lines using state-based modeling. The Journal of Systems and Software 80, 1879–1892 (2007)
17. Méry, D., Singh, N.K.: Functional behavior of a cardiac pacing system. Intern. Journal of Discrete Event Control Systems, IJDECS (2010)
18. Object Management Group: OMG Systems Modeling Language V 1.2 (2010), www.omg.org/spec/SysML/1.2/
19. Schaefer, I., Gurov, D., Soleimanifard, S.: Compositional algorithmic verification of software product lines. In: Aichernig, B.K., de Boer, F.S., Bonsangue, M.M. (eds.) FMCO 2010. LNCS, vol. 6957, pp. 184–203. Springer, Heidelberg (2011)
20. Schobbens, P.Y., Heymans, P., Trigaux, J.C.: Feature diagrams: A survey and a formal semantics. In: Intern. Conf. on Requirements Engineering (RE), pp. 136–145 (2006)
21. Scientific, B.: PACEMAKER System Specification (January 2007)
22. Tuan, Zheng, Tho: Modeling and verification of safety critical systems: A case study on pacemaker. In: 4th Conf. on Secure Software Integration and Reliability Improvement, pp. 23–32. IEEE (2010)
23. Varró, D., Varró, G., Pataricza, A.: Designing the automatic transformation of visual languages. Science of Computer Programming 44(2), 205–227 (2002)

Defining New Structural and Mobile Support to Improve Hospital Facilities Access and Usability

Alessandro Carlini[1,3], Pierluigi Dalla Rosa[2], Bartolomeo Montrucchio[2],
Ivan Cenci[1], Francesca Maria Claudio[1], Giovanni Luongo[1],
Jacopo Spigaroli[1], and Giuseppina Gini[1]

[1] ASP, Politecnico di Milano, piazza L. Da Vinci 32,
Milan, Italy
[2] ASP, Politecnico di Torino, Corso Duca degli Abruzzi 24,
Turin, Italy
[3] University of Bourgogne,
Dijon, France
{pierluigi.dallarosa,ivan.cenci,francesca.claudio,
giovanni.luongo,jacopo.spigaroli}@asp-poli.it,
alessandro.carlini@u-bourgogne.fr,
bartolomeo.montrucchio@polito.it, gini@elet.polimi.it

Abstract. Our target was to improve mobility services within a large hospital center. We considered a modern hospital as case study. Our work had the valuable support of the San Raffaele Hospital (hSR). About patients and visitors' mobility we found vast room for improvement in terms of user-orientation and support to disabled people. We analyzed people flows and service accessibility, to design an integrated mobility support service and generate the final solution. As smartphones provide a countless variety of communication channels, the challenge was the definition of an effective solution for people mobility exploiting these devices. After choosing a location-aware WLAN for tracking Wi-Fi devices, we defined the characteristics of the application for smartphones, and implemented a prototype. Many indexes, such as smartphone adoption growing rates, promising profitability studies, and massive portability of the mobile device indicate a smartphone application as an innovative and valuable support to improve mobility in hospital centers.

Keywords: Hospital areas, mobile services, support for disabled, orientation and navigation.

1   Introduction

The healthcare system is currently facing the challenge of integrating medical care with services able to improving liveability and access to services, for patients and personnel.

The authors had the opportunity to work in the REMEDIA - REinvent MEDIcal Ambient Project, sponsored by the Alta Scuola Politecnica (ASP) school (*www.asp-poli.it*), whose objective was exploring new opportunities to design the "hospital of

J. Weber and I. Perseil (Eds.): FHIES 2012, LNCS 7789, pp. 55–71, 2013.
© Springer-Verlag Berlin Heidelberg 2013

the future", where medical care goes along with liveability and socialization in a technologically-advanced environment.

The medical partner in this project was the San Raffaele Hospital (hSR), an hospital which is actively responding to this challenge creating many services to improve the effectiveness in care and liveableness (a zoo to entertain the youngest patients, pet therapy, shops and bars to make the medical environment more enjoyable, an hotel to give the opportunity to relatives to take care of patients, etc).

Today hospitals are facing new challenges and traditional (continuous) necessities to improve cost-effectiveness and liveability of the proposed services. Beyond the "pragmatic" aspect of the services effectiveness, today every hospital administration has to plan carefully any economical aspect, with more attention than in the past.

This is one of the reasons why today we can notice a reversal trend, toward a unification of distinct facilities. This unification has an important role in charges reduction, and could lead to fewer equipments and brand new performing machines; nevertheless the inevitable consequence of the unification is the increasing in system complexity and the more difficult access to services [4, 9].

The development of the technology field continuously equips us with new tools and –possibly– new solutions. The aim of the present work is to marry these new technologies to the new approaching necessities of the hospital environment.

The first indefeasible duty is the access to services, which mostly consist in the physical access to buildings, structures, rooms. New hospitals are frequently characterized by wide areas and many buildings. As a result, the simple activity of finding the way for a specific ward can become a real challenge for patients and visitors. The problem is further amplified for visually impaired patients, who experience difficulties in reading signs; and to wheelchair users, whose mobility is restricted to particular paths.

In our project we addressed the issues described above, aiming at designing an integrated and innovative mobility support system capable of helping users navigate and reach given places and deliver desired services.

It is important to note that the main objective of the project, i.e. the improvement of the liveability of services offered to users, comes with objectives reflecting other stakeholders' perspectives as well. On the one hand, a hospital needs to guarantee and improve profitability and visibility. On the other hand, several public and private authorities push towards the improvement of the working conditions within hospitals. Following a win-win approach, the present project was developed to meet these different needs and requirement at the same time.

The macro-activities identified as significant, carried out, and described in the following Sections, are:

- Objective focus. In this phase the Team investigated the actual state of "user-oriented" services, and pointed out the opportunity of improving the mobility support service;
- Stakeholders' requirements analysis. Once detailed the scope of the analysis, we worked to elicit Stakeholders' requirements. Particular attention was reserved to patients and visitors, the final users of the service: their requirements were investigated through semi-structured direct interviews;

- Flow analysis. In order to detail the current situation of the hospital mobility service, we analyzed the actual state of patients and visitors' flow within the public areas. The analysis maps the macro-blocks that compose the hospital and the paths connecting them;
- State of the Art analysis. The analysis of best practices in mobility was useful to explore opportunities and generate new ideas. The Team developed a broad investigation, also taking into consideration best practices outside the medical environment but relating to different contexts, as mobility support is an issue that several contexts have in common;
- Generation of new ideas. Thanks to the analysis carried out and leveraging on the academic background, the Team generated new solutions to address the mobility and the access to service issues. Two concepts emerged particularly: the use of Terminal Units (*TU*) and the use of a Smartphone Application (*SA*);
- Valuation and choice of the final solution. The concepts were evaluated according to relevant criteria, namely resolution of users' mobility problems, popularity among users, applicability of the solutions to the different clusters, impact on hospital key requirements and sustainability. Downstream, the *SA* was chosen as the more interesting and advantageous solution to the mobility issue;
- Detailing the final solution. The *SA* was detailed in terms of functionalities, hardware configuration, software deployment, and interface;
- Economical analysis. We developed an "evaluation tool" to support the investment assessment and to estimate benefits in adopting the new solution. The tool was made run with standard hospital data; the outcomes were used to perform a sensitivity analysis on the most critical variables;
- Demonstrator building. The point of arrival is represented by the development of a *SA* able to simulate the navigation along a demonstrative path. It provides information about directions and time to destination, name of the final destination, ads and extra contents.

2   User Requirements

Being this a research for a new solution, the first step necessarily was the identification of the stakeholders; then, their needs and requirements were analyzed and validated.
The identified stakeholders are:

- patients and visitors: all patients receiving treatments in hospital and all people accompanying or visiting such patients;
- hospital personnel: doctors, nurses, et;
- hospital technical area; in our case the Team had the valuable support of the IRIS (Innovation & Research in life and health Services Unit) technical department of the hSR;
- Customer Service, the office responsible for customer relation management.

Other stakeholders identified in the present research, although only indirectly involved in the project, are *Regione Lombardia* and *Ministero della Salute*, respectively the local administration and the ministry of the Italian government addressing public health.

Each stakeholder has specific needs that determine the requirements to be taken into consideration to ensure the success of the project. The needs and requirements were gathered through meetings, and were validated by analyses of the context. In particular, the validation of patients and visitors' requirements was carried out through direct interviews, and subsequent cluster analysis.

The scheme above well fits a "mutually beneficial collaboration" [3], meaning that the problems posed relate more on organizational implementation rather than on conflicts among stakeholders. Indeed, the improvement of the mobility support service meets the main needs of the different stakeholders.

2.1   Interviews

The identification of users' requirements in relation to mobility was carried out through about 30 closed questions, elaborated on the basis of a Fishbone Diagram (Figure. 1).

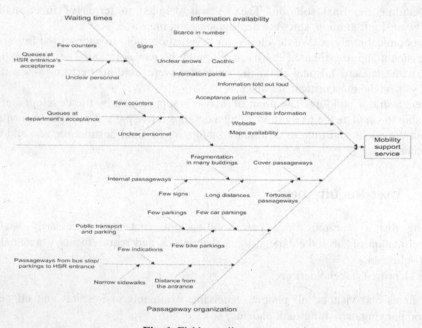

Fig. 1. Fishbone diagram

We interviewed 128 patients and visitors. The interviews, any of which lasted between 15 and 40 minutes, were composed of two parts. The first part consisted in 30 questions with closed answers, aimed to identify the main problems of the users in relation to mobility; the second part was an open-question session aiming to gather the personal insights and suggestions for possible improvements. In the development of both parts the Team was supported by the hSR Customer Service Department.

The answers were classified, normalized, translated in quantitative parameters (where necessary) and analyzed [5]. The analysis was performed through a Pareto approach [8] that allows ranking the problems and defining the priorities of intervention. The main results show the macro-causes of the scarce level of satisfaction towards the mobility support service, namely long waiting times, scarce information, and bad passageways organization.

Following we synthesize the results of the first part of interviews. About information availability the main criticalities are shown in Figure 2; their causes, derived using a Pareto approach, are depicted in Figure 3.

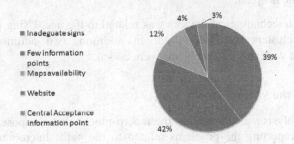

Fig. 2. Pie chart representing an example of the main criticalities and the possible improvements in the current Mobility Support System

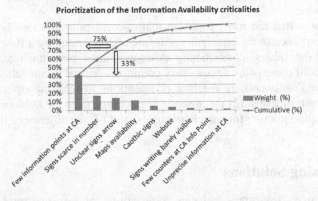

Fig. 3. Third-level causes (with relative weights) of the macro-cause "Information availability", ordered from the most relevant to the least relevant. On the basis of the Pareto law, the arrows underline the dominant causes (CA = Central Acceptance).

Two questions addressed the problem of waiting times. Their analysis showed waiting times at the Central Accepting Office as the "perceived as more relevant" problem; other criticalities are related to the scarceness of parking lots, the distance of no-fee parking, and the path from the parking to the entrance of the structure.

2.2   Cluster Analysis

We explored users' requirements through a Cluster analysis. This analysis is justified by the principle that the totality of patients and visitors is not homogeneous: different typologies are characterized by distinct habits and preferences. Three segmentation criteria were considered predictive to determine the attractiveness of the new solutions:

- How familiar they are with technological devices;
- How familiar they are with hospital structures;
- How they reach the hospital.

The familiarity with technological devices was related to the age. Using these criteria eight significant clusters were identified. In addition, two additional clusters representing people with mobility problems were added.

2.3   Analysis of the Visitors Flow

The aim of this analysis was delineating the macro-blocks that compose the hospital public areas, and reporting the problems related to the paths interconnecting these macro-blocks.

The macro-blocks that generally compose the hospital public area are: (1) wards, (2) reception / acceptance offices, (3) administration offices, (4) arrival points of public transports, (5) car parking; and occasionally: (6) hotels and refectory, (7) education centre.

Results show that the paths from the main access points to the Acceptance, and from the Acceptance to the principal wards, are characterized by a flow density much greater than the others; consequently designers must pay much attention to the characteristics of these paths. Other –very common– critical points (also confirmed by the interviewed' answers) are the lack of attentions to relevant aspects like (1) the excessive length of paths, (2) the absence of coverage over the outdoor paths, (3) the limits of the infrastructure for wheelchair users, and (4) the absence or the unclearness of direction signs.

3   Devising Solutions

Today innovative disciplines and new tools allow for infrastructural improvement providing better visualization of routes and simplification in localization and identification along the path (using colours codes, for example), offering more accessible information to the users by innovative way, and so on.

Considering the present trend, the proposed solution gives priority to the use of innovative digital tools. In particular, on the basis of the requirement analysis, we developed two possible solutions to improve the mobility support within the hospital environment: the use of *TU* and the use of *SA*. The two solutions were analyzed and compared in terms of functionalities, performances, sustainability, adoptability, and compatibility with the current hospital structure. All the details are freely available in the whole report at http://home.dei.polimi.it/gini/ASP/REMEDIA.pdf.

3.1   Terminal Units (*TU* Solution)

The *TU* technology can effectively support the mobility in the hospital areas: the "kiosks" equipped with terminal units can provide a variety of services such as "path-finding" and "map-printing", reducing queues at the information points.

We considered that the main reception represents a very important convergence node. We divided the way towards the wards into two parts: the first encompasses the paths linking the main reception to the three access points, while the second one is represented by the segment which separates the main reception from the wards themselves.

It was evident that users who reach the hospital by bus or place their car in the outer parking have difficulties in finding the way to reach the right hospital ward. Consequently it is necessary to place the *TUs* at least in these areas (i.e. near bus stops, outer and underground parking, ward entrances, etc..).

Seven functionalities were identified for the use of *TUs*.

1. Person Identification
For the access to special services or the diffusion of some information it will be necessary to identify the user. The "Carta regionale dei servizi" could be useful for this purpose.

2. Way Finding
The kiosks could represent an important solution to help people find their way through the hospital structures. In particular, way finding could be supported by a traditional "point to point" navigation system (using more powerful systems like 3D representation and way simulation); or by more effective services, such as user & prescription identification for the automatic path generation, a more readable and "pleasant" interface to help people unfamiliar with technology, destination and path colour code explanation, and so on. The way finding function would let people flow inside the village easier, reducing the routing time to the final destination and improving the effectiveness of hospital services.

3. Booking of Visits/Exams
This function would represent an alternative to the traditional booking channels; this interface (also available through the internet, for example) could display dates and timetable to reserve a visit or an exam, modify a pre-existent condition, or give access to a personal area for more detailed services (i.e. report delivery, report history, vaccinations list, clinic folder, etc.).

4 General Document Printing
As the mobility support and the visits/exams booking, this service and the following (content download, payment, etc) could require the protected user identification.

5 Content Download
Technology-oriented people may find it useful to download contents from the kiosks to their portable devices via wireless connection (e.g. Wifi or Bluetooth). Downloadable contents can be both informative (for example, clinic specialties list) and recreational

6 Payments

The payment function includes the possibility to pay for some services (like parking) and to buy prepaid cards to be used in the bar or shops located inside the hospital village. The payment of services or prepaid cards can be made through *TU* via cash or credit card.

7 Parking Support Service

The main issues related to the parking are two, namely the difficulty to remember where the car is parked, as the parking area is huge, and the cost of parking. The use of *TUs* can help to address these issues: kiosks and parking terminal units could print on the ticket the necessary information to locate the car, and also to pay at the exit.

3.2   Smartphone Application (*SA*)

Smartphones provide phone services, email, multi-protocol wireless communications, PDA capabilities and are now migrating from an embedded architecture to a more distributed and programmable one. These multi-functional phones are becoming an effective new way of dealing with digital technology, as they interact with a hybrid real-virtual environment. Smartphones are accessible to most of the people, are personal and are always in our pocket.

These characteristics show the power of smartphones that is going to grow further in the years to come. Smartphone applications, as presented in the state of the art analysis within medical environment, are already used within hospitals. Indeed, the use of a personal device can help users understand information provided in a more effective way rather than an ad-hoc designed embedded system, although the latter could have a better cognitive interface.

Synthetically, the *SA* can support mobility through guiding the user during all his/her movements within the hospital structure. To do so, the system needs data on user's actual position, final destination and every node inside the hospital. The set of functionalities supported would be:

1 Personal Identification

When booking a visit, either via telephone or on-line, patients register using an account linked to their telephone number. Therefore when they arrive at the hospital and connect to the wireless network through the smartphone, the system automatically recognizes their identity via phone number and provides access and application download. Alternatively, visitors or patients that get to the hospital with a different telephone number from the one associated to their booking can access the services provided connecting to the wireless network manually (i.e. entering their identification data).

2 SMS Alerts

The telephone number is fundamental not only for patient identification, but also for extra services like SMS alerts before the visit. The day before the visit the user receives an SMS reminding him/her of the visit and providing information about how to use the *SA* service. The SMS contains a link to the application, which is downloadable from the internet.

3 Payments

The possibility to pay through the device is really advantageous. Indeed:

- It can optimize queues and reduce people stress;
- It improves sustainability by reducing tickets and receipts printing;
- Discounts for mobile payments can be offered to boost people's use of the Smartphone application.

The use of mobile payments is a strong paradigm-changer because of its new way of looking at money transactions. The user can access mobile payment and use phone credit or credit card to pay for medical services, parking or just having a coffee. People can avoid queues and directly present a digital ticket with a signature that matches up with the transaction. Smartphones often have a good resolution of the screen that allows the use of 2D scanners to read bar-codes on the monitor of phones. When the user pays, the system sends him/her a two-dimensional bar code that will be read when the user needs to show proof of payment for the service.

4 Way finding

The way finding feature, which is the core of the present research and the REMOBILA ASP project, works with three degrees of complexity depending on the choice of the users. Consequently, users could choose within three different visualization modes. First, users can let the smartphone guide them or choose to watch the map where it is shown where they are and the suggested route to destination (if the destination is set). Second, if users are technology-oriented they can choose to interact with the map, other than visualize it. Third, if the user is a patient the application could also show some notes about timing, how much time left before the visit, and an estimation of the time left to destination. The system can manage queues in real-time thanks to the tracking feature. If the patient has problems, he/she can request the help of an operator through the application.

5 General Services

The application could provide some general services too, such as booking online. The SA represents a powerful platform that can be exploited for different purposes. For example, it could be used for ethic marketing, such as sponsoring the donation of the "5x1000" to the hospital, or signalling the presence of bar, shops or other services when searched by the user. What is more, the way to provide messages must be careful planned, in order to respect the environmental and manners rules and the users' tranquillity.

6 Physically Impaired People

About mobility inside a hospital structure, a note about physical impaired people is necessary. We focused on two categories of physical impaired people that could take advantage from the SA:

- People using wheelchairs: the system can recognize their disability thanks to information given during the registration, or can be notified of a temporary wheelchair use by the users themselves. Consequently the system can guide the users along the best route for wheelchairs.
- Visually impaired people: the system can recognize these users in the same way described for people using wheelchairs. Then, a text-to-speech system can drive the

patients, also providing next step and timing information. This support would be useful also for people whose sight is not good enough to read signs or to read the mobile's monitor.

3.3   Solution Evaluation

The evaluation was conducted on the basis of the following criteria:

- *Resolution of users' mobility problems* - The interviews pointed out that the mobility issues are perceived as a priority.

- *Popularity among users* - The interviews conducted not only gathered users' requirements, but also tested the popularity of possible solutions among users, adopting the Co-Creative approach. Answers showed the most appealing solutions to be the *TU* rather than the *SA*.

- *Applicability of the solutions to the different clusters* - Another important criterion of evaluation was the analysis of the clusters supported by the different solutions. Three segmentation criteria were applied: technological attitude, familiarity with the hospital, mean of transportation used to reach the hospital (see paragraph 2.2). The interview outcome showed that the percentage of people appreciating the *SA* solution increases with the decrease of age. It results that Terminal Units are well-adapted to all users, while –today– the *SA* is tailored for users younger than 64. It is important to point out that the number of people supported by the *SA* is doomed to increase in the next years.

- *Impact on hospital key requirements* - Another important criterion is represented by the solution impact on hospital key performances, as illustrated in Section 2. Both solutions guarantee improvements in patients' satisfaction and hospital image, respecting patients' safety. Nevertheless, they are different as far as profitability and privacy are concerned. A preliminary comparative profitability analysis sees the *SA* solution prevail. Indeed, assuming comparable additional revenues, software costs, and interface development costs, the *TU* solution also requires the purchase and the installation of the kiosks, which are generally expensive. On the contrary, the smartphones solution has the advantage of exploiting a device -the smartphone- whose cost has been sustained by users themselves. Smartphones prevail in guaranteeing privacy too. Indeed, each demanded Terminal piece of information can be seen not only by the patient currently using the kiosk, but also by other people passing by. On the contrary, smartphones are strictly personal, guaranteeing privacy.

- *Sustainability* - The comparison between the *TU* and the *SA* solutions leads to the following considerations. While mobility is supported by the kiosks through the possibility of printing the path to follow, the *SA* provides all the information on the display of the device. Therefore, smartphones allow eliminating the paper depletion implied in the usage of the terminals. Furthermore, the use of smartphones enables mobile payment, that further reduces paper waste (given by tickets, receipts etc.). Finally, the *TU* solution requires the installation of several kiosks within the hospital, which implies high levels of resource consumption both for the production phase and for the operating phase. On the other hand, the *SA* adds functionalities to a device that is already owned by users, so that additional resources depletion for producing and operating the devices are eliminated. Summing up, the comparison between the two solutions sees *SA* to prevail.

In conclusion, the Smartphone device appears as better supporting the user mobility and the service depletion. The device is purchased by the owner in reason of other personal uses/benefits; the confidentiality of information, as well as identification and customization, are a natural consequence "by design". The "portability" of information and services is at the maximum value (the device is following the person, where for the "totem" solution we obtain the opposite condition). Finally, the present availability of services and software assisting peoples with handicaps (e.g. TTS, Screenreader, voice control and dictation input, "Ray Phone", "Fifth Sens", "VizWiz", etc.) suggests the Smartphone-based solution as the more egalitarian and by consequence the finest.

4   The Profitability Analysis

Profitability represents a fundamental requirement. For this reason the financial impact of the solution was studied associating strategic impacts (e.g. increased mobility service level) and main actions (e.g. purchase and installation of infrastructures) to the financial dimensions (i.e. revenues or costs) they have an impact on. The analysis was based on the evaluation of some profitability indexes, namely Net Present Value and Payback Time. Nevertheless, some differences arose with respect to the standard evaluation process [6, 10].

Therefore, an "evaluation tool" was developed. This tool, built on the basis of the analysis of revenue and cost drivers of the project, could be used by any hospital partner for a more precise evaluation of the investment. It has a general validity, and it supports the evaluation of the *SA* solution in wide range of contexts. What is more, the tool was also used to perform a sensitivity analysis on critical variables. Main results are presented hereafter.

The first step of the economic analysis for the *SA* was the translation of strategic impacts into financial impacts [1], as illustrated in Figure 4.

The following feasibility analysis studied main financial impacts, reasoning in differential terms from the actual state case.

The new mobility solution is expected to have a positive impact on hospital revenues, given by the increase in the mobility Service Level (SL) and the ethic proximity marketing. As a result, the total additional revenues per user of the *SA* can be calculated as in Eq 1:

$$\Delta R = \Delta R_{fromCoreActivityPerPerson} * \text{Num-users} + \Delta R_{fromMarketingActivities} \qquad (1)$$

where ΔR, the total additional revenues, is given from the sum of the additional revenues from person related health services times the Num-users (= number of users adopting the smartphone solution) and the additional revenues related to additional services (not health related).

A fundamental revenue driver is the number of users adopting the solution. The main parameters that influence this number are:

- number of persons in need of mobility support that go to hospital per day.
- percentage of smartphones in Italy (nowadays around the 25% of phones);
- adoption rate of the new solution by patients and visitors. A conservative value for this parameter, suggested by hSR, is 3%. The internal variables that would influence this number are: effectiveness of the interface, accessibility to impaired people and "Service Level" perceived by users.

Therefore, the total number of users (including in and out patients and visitors) in the year t is calculated as in Eq 2:

$$\text{Users}^t = \text{Num-people} * \%\text{peopleNeedingMobilitySupport} * \text{Adoption.rate} *$$
$$(\text{Adoption-rate-growth})^t \tag{2}$$

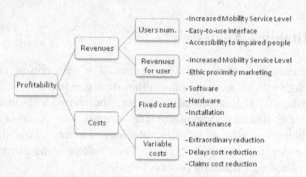

Fig. 4. Transposition of the strategic impact into the financial impact

About costs estimation, we observed that the main impact of the solution would be an increase in efficiency, reducing the cost per person if he/she adopts the solution. Cost efficiencies, which increase with the number of users, would be given by:

- extra hours cost reduction (the new solution would reduce visits delays);
- claims cost reduction (traditionally people experiencing delays result in both image costs and a out-of-pocket costs, like reimbursements and similar);
- delays cost reduction (out-of-pocket costs, such as unexploited machinery activation, unused solution preparation, and similar).

The solution is also associated to additional cost entries, concerning new hardware, software, installation, and training (we detailed and evaluated a possible package; in the present article we avoid to present specific solutions and commercial brands).

5   Final Design and Demonstrator Implementation

5.1   Choice between "Intelligence" Located on the Client or Server Side

The first decision taken was whether to put the "intelligence" (i.e. main database and main elaboration) on the client side or server side. In both cases the user, who owns a smartphone, has to register online - typically at home; then when arriving at the hospital he/she can access information previously downloaded, or may receive networked information. In the client side approach the smartphone is aware of the location of the patient and it is also responsible for location discovery, route calculation and identification. The knowledge of the structure is embedded in the client so the user can simply open the service on the smartphone, enabling it to show information. Using a server to process all the requests about way finding can be more complex but the hospital could have some extra benefits: more control on the system, awareness of the position of users in real-time and possibility to give users only the information they need. The server-side intelligence solution appears to be the most interesting; it guarantees a wide accessibility and a lighter client-side burden. Therefore this model is considered to be the most convenient to develop.

5.2   Designing the Infrastructure

The standard solutions exploiting GPS signals are not sustainable due to the lack of GPS coverage in indoor areas. To support the smartphone location the installation of a location-aware WLAN might be sufficient; this structure might also satisfy other hospital needs nowadays emerging, such as asset tracking, or providing different and new services to the patients.

We found, on the commercial market, systems able to track up to 2500 devices simultaneously, a number in line with the visitors to a modern extended hospital (we verified the presence of other systems with more powerful performances as well).

The chosen system [2] uses a distance-based technique (lateration) to discriminate the position of the mobile device by using received signal strength (RSS) measured by at least 3 access points surrounding it. Proper placement of access points should be respected in order to exploit the full performance potential of the system. Antennas should be mounted such that they have a clear 360° view, without being blocked at close range by large objects. The distance between deployed access points can have an impact on location performance, as well as the performance of co-resident voice and data applications.

In our pilot study, we considered the criticalities of paths in the hospital and we dimensioned the system accordingly (Figure 5).

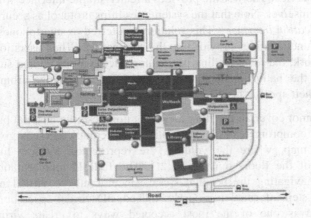

Fig. 5. An example of deployment of the access points

The WLAN infrastructure allows the installation of third-party location clients to reside in the Unified Wireless Network in a complementary fashion to Wireless Control System (WCS), or in substitution to it. WCS is meant to keep track of every device located in the controlled area, but does not send this information to the objects tracked. For this reason it is needed an additional location client with the duty of notifying each single smartphone of its own position. Besides the plain sending of the position to the tracked device, according to the "Server-Side Intelligence" philosophy the system has to calculate the route from the current position to the destination and send it to the smartphone. Finally, an ad-hoc SW installed on the smartphone has the task of showing this information and managing the interaction with the user.

5.3   Designing the Software Application

The point of arrival of the project is represented by the development of a software application to be installed on a smartphone that simulates the navigation along a demonstrative path. In this context, the user interface should guarantee the most clear and quick access to the functions of the application. The demonstrator mainly consists in the elaboration of the mobile application interface, which is a key element in determining the success or the failure of the solution. We developed different interfaces [11] for the different clusters of users identified.

Two alternative scenarios were taken into consideration: smartphone models that do not support native applications and smartphone models that support native application.

- *Web-based location system interface* - This solution is referred to smartphones that have access limitations, due to the API provided by common browsers and poor performance of non compiled code. For these smartphones we developed a simplified solution based on the access to services via browser. When the user joins the hospital wireless network, the main landing page could automatically pop up and open the hospital web service. The website provides a really simple interface where users have to identify themselves. Note that the system uses https protocol as security measure.

- *Native application interface* - This solution is referred to smartphones that have full access to all functionalities provided by the application. When users join the hospital wireless network, the main landing page automatically pops up and supplies the link to download the native application. Its interface can change from user to user according to their specific needs and aptitudes.

A 2D map cannot cover all the floor areas that compose the hospital buildings at one sight. A good compromise between simplicity and completeness is given by a really essential 3D map, where the volumes are represented by few lines while the visualization of the floors remains in 2D. The full-3D representation is the best solution for navigating the hospital space, since it allows virtual navigation and supports next step information properly. Indeed, 3D virtual space combined with a camera model is one of the most accepted ways to create virtual interactive environments [7].

On the basis of the above considerations, we developed and prototyped three different solutions, selectable from the home page: (1) next move information, (2) 2D map, and (3) 3D map. The three associated icons are located in the home page in an effective way. In western culture, attention focuses first on the top-left corner of the screen, and then jumps to the areas with the biggest characters. The easiest navigation modality view, targeted to non-digital natives, has hence to be located where the attention focuses (top-left corner) and is associated to a graphic icon. The three modalities, illustrated in Figure 6, are detailed as follows:

Simplified Navigation view - It shows essential information only, i.e. next step from current position to next node. This kind of interface can be used with headphones too, thanks to a text-to-speech software agent. Consequently, it is suitable for people that prefer audio indication and, more important, for visually impaired people and wheelchair users. We consider that wheelchair users would be facilitated by the use of headphones because it guarantees the possibility to free their hands.

2D Navigation view - This view gives access to the 2D map. Through it, it is possible to see an overview of the whole path from the current position to the final destination, and to search for places of interest. The application highlights the places of interest in relation to the user condition. This view is also useful when leaving the hospital, as the "park button" could guide the user to the car.

3D Navigation view - This last view is the most complex, since the application shows a 3D visualization of the whole hospital structure. Users can navigate the 3D map with the typical gestures of interaction in mobile applications (e.g. tapping).

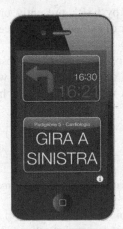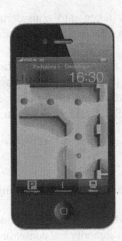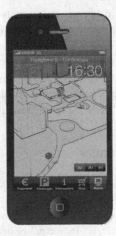

Fig. 6. The three interfaces for path finding

6   Conclusions

REMEDIA project has been a remarkable example of synergic work, where the harmonization of different expertises (engineering, management, and architecture) of the team members has permitted the success of the project, combining media-oriented interfaces, architectural reproductions of hospital buildings, and studies of technical and economical feasibility. The outcome of this collaboration is the design of the Smartphone Application (*SA*) for guiding users, which is a novel interpretation of the mobility support in which technology represents an important but not fundamental tool.

Indeed, the most challenging task to be faced nowadays is not the development of the technology, which has reached remarkably high levels, but its adequate use in relation to users' needs. To do so, hospital users' interviews were of extreme value, providing requirement insight for the final solution. A strong contribution was also given by the evaluation of the actual state of patients and visitors and the flow within the hospital public areas, which allowed us to spot the problems related to the outer hospital paths.

Translating the theoretical design of the solution into an implementable concept was an interesting and challenging task. We chose wireless triangulation for the assessment of smartphones location, dimensioned the infrastructure in terms of access points and proposed a break-even implementation approach. With regard to the feasibility of the solution, we developed an "evaluation tool" to be used by the hospital for the precise evaluation of the investment. Finally we developed a software application to be installed on smartphones that simulates the navigation along a demonstrative path, including a variety of navigation modalities tailored to different segments.

The designed solution is now taken into consideration by hSRl, presently under huge management transformation, and definitively in favour of extending e-services.

Acknowledgments. The authors acknowledge the Alta Scuola Politecnica for hosting their REMEDIA Project, aimed at designing the "hospital of the future". The work would not have been possible without the strong interaction with Alberto Sanna, head of the "IRIS" Scientific Institute San Raffaele in Milan.

References

1. Azzone, G., Bertelè, U.: Valutare l'innovazione. Analisi e controllo degli investi-menti. Etaslibri, Italy (1998)
2. Cisco Systems Inc.: Enterprise Mobility 4.1 Design Guide, San Josè, CA, USA (2009).
3. Dente, B.: Public policy between authority and consensus – private communication (2011)
4. Hospital Build Asia 2011 Exibition & Congress, Marina Bay Sands, Singapore (2011)
5. Ishikawa, K.: Cause and effect diagram. In: Proceedings International Conference on Quality Control, Tokyo, Japan, pp. 607–610 (1963)
6. Jovanovic, P.: Application of sensitivity analysis in investment project evaluation under uncertainty and risk. International Journal of Project Management 17, 217–222 (1999)

7. Manovich, L.: The Language of New Media. MIT Press, Cambridge (2001)
8. Mathur, V.K.: How Well Do We Know Pareto Optimality? How Well Do We Know Pareto Optimality? Journal of Economic Education 22(2), 172–178 (1991)
9. Optimizing Patient Flow: Moving Patients Smoothly Through Acute Care Settings. IHI Innovation Series white paper. Institute for Healthcare Improvement, Boston (2003)
10. Pindyck, R.S.: Irreversibility, Uncertainty, and Investment. Journal of Economic Literature 29(3), 1110–1148 (1999)
11. Raskin, J.: The Humane Interface: New Directions for Designing Interactive System. Addison Wesley (2000)

Regulated Software Development –
An Onerous Transformation

Oisín Cawley[1,*], Xiaofeng Wang[2], and Ita Richardson[1]

[1] Lero-The Irish Software Engineering Research Centre,
University of Limerick, Ireland
{Oisin.Cawley,Ita.Richardson}@lero.ie
[2] Free University of Bozen
Bolzano, Italy
xiaofeng.wang@unibz.it

Abstract. Software development within regulated settings is becoming more and more common place. Compliance typically involves saying what you do and doing what you say. However, in some domains, especially safety-critical ones, it needs to be more than simply following the rules, and should be something which everybody in the organisation supports in their daily tasks. This can be difficult to achieve and requires an organisational transformation, but once begun, sets the foundation on which the software development process can evolve.

Keywords: Regulated Industry Standards, Software Process, Software Quality, Medical Information Systems.

1   Introduction

Many years ago there was an advertisement on Television which went something like, "If you had the only car in the world, you could drive where you like, but you haven't so you can't". It was obviously a road safety commercial to re-enforce acceptable rules of driving, but this is very similar to what we are experiencing in the world of regulated software development today. If your application was the only software running, with no interaction with other systems, and no possible effect on third parties then who cares how you develop it?

However, this is not the case for an increasing number of companies. Industries such as the financial services, safety-critical domains like aviation and medical devices, and companies listed on the U.S. stock exchange have seen the conditions under which they operate change significantly in recent times. These changes have affected the software development processes within such companies by introducing software compliance rules. These additional requirements may take various forms depending on the type of regulations which apply. What is important to know is that they introduce some significant changes which not only can be time consuming and

---

* Corresponding author.

J. Weber and I. Perseil (Eds.): FHIES 2012, LNCS 7789, pp. 72–86, 2013.
© Springer-Verlag Berlin Heidelberg 2013

expensive for the software development teams, but have a wide affect within the broader organisation.

Our research has shown that the process changes which must be introduced to satisfy the regulations, transform peoples' daily activities and therefore need to be given the attention and care due of any transformation process. The focus or intention of the regulations is important. A clear understanding of this will drive: the design of your new development processes, where a concentrated change management process will be needed, and the type and level of detailed evidence to be maintained for those crucial and sometimes painful audits.

2 Research Process

In this paper we have drawn on research into regulated software development from both a financial and safety-critical perspective.

One author has 11 years experience working in a large US multinational (MyOrg) (Cawley and Richardson, 2010), and 7 of those under the Sarbanes-Oxley (SOX) regulations (www.soxlaw.com). MyOrg is a leader in global supply chain business process management. NASDAQ listed, it has over 25 centres in 14 countries and has a diverse and interconnected collection of information systems which are developed and maintained by a combination of in-house and outsourced personnel. By means of reflective analysis we examined the effects on the software development and support teams when the SOX regulations came into effect in 2002.

With a growing interest in modern software development methodologies (SDMs) such as Agile and Lean, we performed a mapping study of these SDMs within safety-critical regulated domains (Cawley et al., 2010). The resulting state-of-the-art gave us a solid understanding of the development issues in such domains as Aviation, Automotive, and Medical Devices.

The Medical Device industry is seen as a growth area in many countries, and is fast developing into a race for world leadership. As an industry, which was somewhat immune to cost pressures, it is now feeling the effect of the demand for lower cost products. By means of an in-depth case study at a medical device manufacturing plant (MedTech), we examined the issues affecting the software development and which typically lead to the adoption of heavy SDMs (Cawley et al., 2011). MedTech is a US multinational with over 25,000 employees and develops medical solutions. A series of semi-structured interviews brought to light the concerns people had with the software development life-cycle (SDLC) and how the regulations had impacted it.

We have synthesised this data into a model of influences which is presented in this paper.

3 The Effects of Compliance

The SDLC within a regulated area is reflective of a number of key influences. We synthesised our findings into a common model, categorising the influences into 4 groups. These categories together with some of their main influences are depicted in Figure 1, with a selection of exemplars included for each.

3.1   Regulations

At the top of Figure 1 we have the first of these contextual elements, regulations. Why do we have regulations and how important are they in terms of the development of medical device software? According to (Campbell, 2004), regulations are simply a form of social organisation, and therefore supports the definition of regulations used in this study as being: "*rules, principles, or conditions that govern procedure or behaviour*" (The-Free-Dictionary, 2011). There are those who argue that there is too much regulation and that not enough research has been done in assessing the adequacy of regulations in achieving their intended aims (Campbell, 2004). For example, regulations governing financial institutions, such as the Basel Accord (Basel, 2004) and the Sarbanes-Oxley Act (SOX, 2002), did not prevent the global banking crises of 2007.

There are, however, different types or levels of regulation ranging from low (self regulation), medium (Government regulation), to high (Litigation) (Bush, 2007). It is only when a lower form of regulation is seen to be ineffective is it raised to a higher level. Nonetheless, it is difficult to argue against high levels of regulation which aim to ensure human safety. For example, the standards and recommended practices issued by the Association for the Advancement of Medical Instrumentation (AAMI), aspire to a "*continued increase in the safe and effective application of current technologies to patient care*" (ANSI/AAMI/IEC, 2006), a laudable objective. While there is little debate about the merit of such motives, the AAMI does however have an additional objective, namely "*the encouragement of new technologies*" (Ibid). There is therefore a balance which needs to be struck between this drive for innovation and need for a high degree of device safety and the consequent higher level of regulation (Ziegler, 2006).

Other safety-critical domains such as automotive, aviation, and nuclear have similar concerns when it comes to human safety. However, the domains differ with respect to the governing regulations. Given the technical specialisation of each area, this is not surprising. There is a consequent need to tailor development activities such as risk management for the specific domain in which the systems are deployed. For example, MDs govern a wide range of products including many which will be operated by the patient themselves.

Each country has its own specific regulatory requirements when it comes to medical device software. Within the United States it is governed by the Code of Federal Regulations Title 21. Within the European Union (E.U.) it is the Medical Devices Directive. More and more, such federal documents are allowing for adherence to international standards such as (ISO, 2003, ISO, 2007, ANSI/AAMI/IEC, 2006), to satisfy these requirements. It is the influences, affected by such international standards and guidelines, which make the medical device software development process unique. Our research has found that medical device companies predominantly employ what can be described as heavy weight software development methodologies to ensure all required steps are taken to satisfy regulatory requirements.

Within our model, the arrows emanating from the Regulations box are shown leading to the other three categories, indicating that compliance with the regulations must be addressed within multiple levels and contexts.

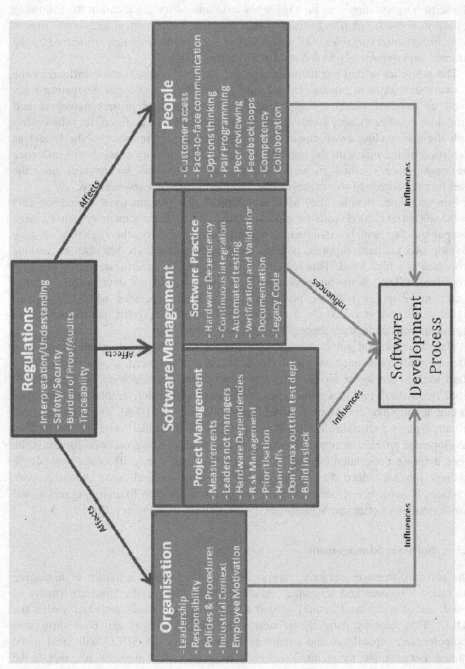

Fig. 1. Categories of Influences on the SDLC within a Regulated Context

3.2   Organisation

The term 'Organisation' can be a nebulous term and so for clarification the following definition is used: "*[An] organisation is a complex social system and is the sum of many interrelated variables. The operations of the organisation are influenced by the external environment of which it is part*" (Mullins, 2004).

The relevance within our theoretical model is that the organisation influences the software development process by defining development tasks and delegating roles (such as developers and testers), responsibilities (such as project managers and validation engineers), and authority (such as approvals). In addition, its relationship with the surrounding environment is an important aspect relevant to the model as identified by the link with the regulations box. The regulatory context will influence the organisation's ethos in terms of ensuring safe and secure software, the workforce's attitude to risk management, and their sense of responsibility.

For example, within the MD regulations, the international standard ISO 13485:2003 (ISO, 2003) calls for a documented quality management system. In large companies, that will be satisfied at multiple levels. Firstly, the organisation may develop and publish corporate policies and procedures which describe the various processes at a high level. This is then complemented by specific standard operating procedures (SOPs) at the business unit level, and/or a software development process documents detailing software practices. Lower level processes which align with higher level ones demonstrate a coherent and unified approach, across the whole organisation, to addressing the regulatory requirements.

The organisational guidelines and supports for the software development process often require significant investment. To protect that investment, an organisation will often seek to employ a formal software development methodology which is future proof (teachable), provides consistency, generates explicit deliverables, and provides an engineering-like development discipline (Roberts et al., 1998). The organisational influence plays a crucial role when it comes to the implementation of such a software development process or implementing changes to an existing process, for example, when entering a regulated industry. Such process changes may affect the way people do their jobs or indeed the job descriptions themselves, and since changing work practices is not a trivial undertaking, it should be dealt with like any organisational transformation (Kotter and Schlesinger, 1979), (Small and Downey, 2001).

3.3   Software Management

The software management box incorporates the overlapping activities of managing the tasks, resources and schedules, combined with the specific practices (many of which are of a technical nature) needed to perform the various activities within the SDLC. This category naturally influences the SDLC since it will be within these competencies, capabilities and situational contexts that the SDLC will need to be framed. For example, the technical nature of the product will automatically dictate the type of skills required and the type of development environment needed. The availability or lack or availability of these resources will shape the resulting SDLC (Kettunen and Laanti, 2005). In addition, the existing technical infrastructure will go some way towards assisting or hindering the adoption of a specific SDLC approach. For example a company which uses a language not conducive to an object oriented approach (Poppendieck and Poppendieck, 2003) (such as earlier versions of Visual basic, Fortran and Pascal), may have difficulty in following an SDLC which calls for such practices. Similarly, unless some investment is made in additional hardware and/or software, an SDLC which promotes test driven development (Beck, 2002) and continuous integration (Hibbs et al., 2009) is unlikely to be proposed where the environment is not adequately equipped.

Within the domain of MD software, there is an inherent risk to human safety. Consequently, the industry employs various techniques to reduce this risk of harm. Similar to other safety-critical domains, techniques such as Fault Tree Analysis, Failure Mode and Effects Analysis, Failure Mode Effects and Criticality Analysis serve to assist in identifying possible faults, their criticality and the probability of their occurrence. However, specific to the MD domain are the regulations as defined in ISO 14971 (Application of risk management to medical devices) (ISO, 2007) and IEC 62304 (Medical Device Software life cycle processes) (ANSI/AAMI/IEC, 2006). These standards lay down the requirements for ensuring that risk management (RM) is appropriately catered for within the SDLC. By assigning each software system a software safety class, the manufacturer can use it as a guide to the specific processes and tasks that are needed as part of their development process.

Different people and organisations approach project management of software development differently. Depending on the perceived importance of the software, for example is it seen as a strategic competitive advantage (Porter, 1998), (Prahalad and Hamel, 1990), or merely an asset to be managed (Ben-Menachem, 2008), (OECD, 2011), the SDLC will reflect this. A company which sees the software as being strategically important may also be more supportive of pursuing lean or agile approaches such as iterative development (Rasmussen et al., 2009) and/or closer contact between developers and end users (Rottier and Rodrigues, 2008) in order to improve that key process area.

3.4   People

An obvious influence on the software development process are the people who are involved with it on a daily basis. There are a myriad of areas which have been studied over the years surrounding the issues with software development due to the human condition. For example the fundamental problems associated with knowledge management in such a specialist environment continues right up to the present day (Robillard, 1999), (Damian and Zowghi, 2002), (Ye et al., 2008), (Levy and Hazzan, 2009). Another factor is the motivation of the software developers themselves (Burn et al., 1991), (Sharp and Hall, 2009), (Treude et al., 2011), something considered to be the most impactful on productivity (Boehm, 1981). Indeed unmotivated developers can be seen as sources of negative productivity and a liability to a project's success (McConnell, 1998).

The effect of regulatory compliance is very notable at a personnel level as it is precisely the human activities that are being governed. When moving from an unregulated into a regulated environment, unless the work processes are already fulfilling the regulations (experience suggests that this is unlikely), there is a need for peoples' daily activities to change. For example, both SOX and MD regulations look for some level of independence in certain key areas. SOX looks for segregation of duties when it comes to code deployment or even access to a production system, while MD regulations expect independence between developers and validation engineers. The typical approaches to activities such as communication and knowledge transfer, where important ad hoc conversations go undocumented, or an approval is given verbally, are no longer acceptable. When people are used to operating in an environment where issues can be fixed "on the spot", these tighter controls can be very frustrating for both the technical employee as well as for the person awaiting resolution.

4   A Transformation Process

In 2007 the European Medical Device Directive (MDD) expanded its definition of a MD to include stand alone software in its own right to be a possible MD (McHugh et al., 2011). As was the case when SOX was enacted in 2002, this is where a transformation process will be necessary. In other words, existing processes and work habits need to change, and as with any change process requires disciplined attention to some important aspects (Small and Downey, 2001).

This transformation is not only a change in physical activities such as recording test results or maintaining traceability, but equally requires a change in mindset. For example, the MD regulations hold risk management (RM) (safety risk as opposed to, for example, project risk) as a critical aspect of the product development:

> *"The manufacturer shall establish, document and maintain throughout the life-cycle an ongoing process for identifying hazards associated with a medical device, estimating and evaluating the associated risks, controlling these risks, and monitoring the effectiveness of the controls"* (ISO, 2003).

The words "throughout the life-cycle an ongoing process" means it is not something that starts and finishes during a particular phase of the life-cycle but is something that must be woven into the entire process. From a software point of view, RM is completely irrelevant without the context of the surrounding device or people and processes. A software failure alone cannot cause harm. It is important therefore that the interface between the software team and other teams, such as the hardware developers and quality engineers, supports an ethos of thinking about hazards in a cross functional holistic sense at all times (Figure 2).

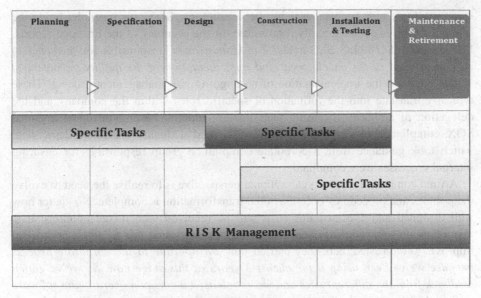

Fig. 2. SDLC with RM across the entire process

In order to structure the discussion around such a transformation we utilise the four categories identified in Figure 1 and draw on specific examples for clarity.

4.1 Organisation

Changing work practices, in order to be compliant, requires the generation of a sense of urgency typical of a transformation process (Kotter, 1995). However, if this urgency is not communicated in a timely manner, it can lead to severe teething problems when it comes to being audited. Within MyOrg, the first dry-run SOX audit presented some non-conformances because there was no evidence of compliance dating back to the official launch date. Although evidence could be collected from dates after this, the issue resulted in a painful retrospective evidence gathering exercise.

Similarly, within the MD regulations, ISO 13485:2003 (ISO, 2003) states that management has the responsibility of "*communicating to the organisation the importance of meeting customer as well as statutory regulatory requirements*". MedTech's approach to this was to develop a mandatory training schedule for all employees on the newly formed product development process, administered by the human resources department.

Leadership is an important attribute in a transformation process. Especially within larger organisations, the need for a strong guiding hand is required (Kotter, 1995). This need manifests itself at a number of levels, however, certain important roles and responsibilities will be mandated by the regulations. SOX, for example, holds the senior executives as individually responsible for the accuracy of the financial reports. MD standard ISO 13485:2003 holds *"Top Management"* responsible for *"evidence of its commitment to the development and implementation of the quality management system"* and for the implementation of an ongoing risk management process. These typically translate into the formation of specific roles within the company and the delegation of authority to ensure their implementation. MyOrg instituted a global SOX compliance officer, while MedTech formed a quality assurance department which took guidance from a corporate compliance group responsible for ensuring internal processes were compliant.

A final comment from an organisational perspective is to realise the need to evolve the policies and procedures once the initial transformation is complete. No matter how well designed and executed this is, it will be received with mixed opinions. It is incumbent on senior management to be aware of and solicit this feedback in order to improve. Within MedTech, they carried out *"an upgrade to the corporate process because we've been using it for almost 3 years at this stage now. So we've gotten feedback from the different sites and we've released a common overarching software policy that governs the whole corporation"* (a senior software quality engineer). Similarly, within MyOrg, they reviewed the processes internally one year after SOX was introduced, leading to a revision of the process documents, thus reducing the associated overheads.

4.1.1 The Bottom Line

If the focus of a organisation is to make money (Goldratt, 1992), then the cost of operations is a critical concern. Compliance costs money. These costs come in many forms, such as employee training, longer project timelines, additional verification & validation (V&V), audits (internal and external), data archiving and staying on top of regulatory updates. Within MyOrg, the software development group automatically added 20% to project estimates to account for the extra activities. This reduced as time went on and processes got more embedded in daily activities but from a business management point of view caused some alarm as project costs jumped. MedTech had a similar experience which led to many projects not proceeding at all.

The requirements around V&V, for example within the MD regulations, in addition to adding cost, also cause confusion. The confusion resides with the regulatory documents, in that they are necessarily broad based and unspecific in terms of how V&V should be performed (Vogel, 2010). In fact this is a common criticism of the regulatory documents in general: *"I think the regulations haven't reached full maturity in terms of what's needed. Certainly the FDA regulations, the actual text of it, is a couple of paragraphs. A lot of it is interpretation after that"* (Senior Engineer, MedTech). Because of this lack of clarity and the risk averse nature of the business units, there is a tendency to do too much in order to be compliant. Speaking about their validation process, a MedTech project leader said *"Personally I think we over club it a lot of the time"*. Not only can the physical validation be overdone, but the documentary evidence required around it generates a lot of concern: *"We're caught in this deadlock of paperwork... The physical work is costing me X, and 3 to 4X is what it's costing me to actually fill out the paper work to validate it"*.

While cost pressures continue to increase, this additional cost is an unwelcome burden. However, this reality needs to be reflected in the expectations of the business management teams. It also behoves the software development teams to find ways to streamline these new tasks to minimise cost. The following exemplifies the point: *"Since [the process introduction] we've been looking and going, 'Oh my God', this has nearly crippled the business, we need to Lean it and take it all back out again"* (Principle Engineer, MedTech). Software development techniques, such as test driven development, automated testing, continuous integration, and automatic document generation can aid in simplifying the processes. They can support finding and eliminating defects as early as possible, and can also help ease the transformation process by implementing a more lean and agile approach (Cawley et al., 2011).

4.2   Software Management

Depending on the industry, the regulations will have different levels of tolerance to compliance. Moving from unregulated to regulated requires an understanding of that level of tolerance. Within the MD domain, for example, there is little tolerance when it comes to demonstrating compliance *"If you're Microsoft you can release something that has a tolerable quality level but it still has problems with it. Whereas in our environment it's a lot more, you cannot go any further until you have done this. You must tick 100% of the boxes not 95% or 80%"* (MedTech Senior Engineer). Within safety-critical companies, management therefore have little appetite when it comes to changing established processes for fear of falling foul of the regulators. Nevertheless, the modern business environment is calling for more efficient and cost effective processes, and so change is inevitable.

To ensure compliance, a common approach to software project management is a phase-gate process. The salient point is the identification of specific development phases with clearly defined entry and exit criteria. Only when these criteria have been fulfilled can you enter/progress to the next stage. This approach seems to be a consequence of the regulations *"The regulations have driven us, or the interpretation of the regulations have driven us towards meeting particular gates or milestones or particular steps"* (MedTech Senior Engineer).

The regulations, however, do not prescribe any particular methodology, even though they may look and read like they favour such a waterfall-type approach. For example, ISO14971:2007 (ISO, 2007) states that "This standard does not require a particular software development life-cycle". What this allows for then, is the potential to evolve the development process and look at more efficient approaches. Our research has seen that companies are looking to the advantages that might be gained from agile methodologies such as eXtreme Programming (XP) and Scrum and, consequently, finding the evolution of their SDLC less problematic than anticipated (Cawley et al., 2010).

Evolving your company's software development process, typical in un-regulated industries, should be no different within regulated domains. In fact, we would suggest that the influences of the regulations lead to the adoption of inefficient development processes. This can be attributed to a lack of clarity/understanding and fear of non-compliance. Once the initial process transformation occurs and becomes embedded, we suggest that companies will start finding weaknesses and will need to adjust their software processes accordingly. These changes will be in many forms such as more effective resource scheduling or implementing lean and agile practices. Within MedTech, they reduced the time for a typical validation process by 30%: "*When we started out, there were validations that were effectively ongoing for 6, 9 months that just got bogged down and ran into problems ... now we were saying we're going to do this and we're going to complete it in 3 months*". By realising that resources were being inefficiently scheduled, they examined ways to address it, such as load levelling. Similar to the Kanban system in lean manufacturing (Anderson, 2010) and using cards to represent different activities within the software project, they identified where bottlenecks were occurring: "*The card represents something, so in my case it was representing a validation protocol or validation execution*" (MedTech, Senior Engineer). By making the issues visible it was easier to discuss and address them "*It was a bit like clearing the jam in the pipe. Once you got them moving you got a big flow, it made a big difference*".

In addition, being a little less dogmatic when it came to fully completing documentation, allowed them to achieve faster prototype systems without breaching regulations: "*... we discovered through pain that we need to give them a piece of equipment and let them run it for a while and they come back and tell you what they actually really want*".

4.3   People

An organisation can't change unless its people change (Mathiassen et al., 2005). One way to achieve this is to issue new SOPs for project activities. Before rolling these out, however, it is important for employees to be brought up to speed on why there is a need for change and how the new SOPs satisfy that need. If this is not clearly enunciated then people may look for shortcuts. As a software developer at MedTech put it: "*Before, we thought the system wasn't great and this [the new process] came along which probably was worse. I don't know how this came about*". This lack of clarity/buy in can result in short cutting or working outside the defined process: "*You find that there's an awful lot of background work done before we start the development proper...We officially don't know about that*" (Senior Software Quality Engineer, MedTech).

A further difficulty with transforming work practices is coping with legacy systems. Older products, developed using previous processes and practices, may not be suitably designed or have available the requisite artefacts to suit the new process. In this case, software modifications may have to be performed differently depending on the project. In addition, if an employee is assigned only to such legacy systems, then, despite having been fully trained, they get very little exposure to the new processes and are potential liabilities if assigned to projects using the new approach. As stated by a MedTech software developer about the new process: *"It's 2 years here in [MedTech] that they've started doing it. I actually haven't worked on a project yet, in the development phase that has used it"*.

Transforming employee work practices is therefore a protracted affair and requires careful implementation and monitoring until the practices start to get embedded: *"Once you get to know what you need, and the order of things, after that period of time it becomes second nature"* (MedTech Software Developer).

5   Discussion and Recommendations

Regulatory compliance from a software development perspective can be daunting for a company which is unfamiliar with it. The effects of regulation are widespread within an organisation and, due to the inexact nature of the regulatory documents, compliance can lead to inefficient and heavy development lifecycles.

This of course does not have to be the case. It is important to really understand the intention of the regulations, and once that is crystal clear, define the processes accordingly. We should remember that the people best suited to determining how to achieve the objectives of the regulations are the people who work in these specific contexts.

Each company is different and so a one-size-fits-all approach will not work. Rolling out an umbrella policy or procedure across an entire organisation will lead to inefficient work practices. Even within companies, different departments will need to have flexibility in how they shape their processes. For example, the research and development department needs to be free to innovate without getting bogged down in red tape. In addition, because the software development process is a collaborative process, the overlapping between departments needs to be smooth.

We should remember that many of the activities mandated by the regulations are probably already being performed to some degree. There is nothing ground breaking in what they look for, just a more robust method of ensuring the right things are happening. Becoming compliant therefore requires a careful transformation process which takes a multi-layered view. Once this initial transformation effort happens, the way is paved for an improvement process which evolves the SDLC.

We conclude with a series of recommended steps, shown in Figure 3, which can assist the successful introduction of regulatory compliant software development processes within a medical device organisation.

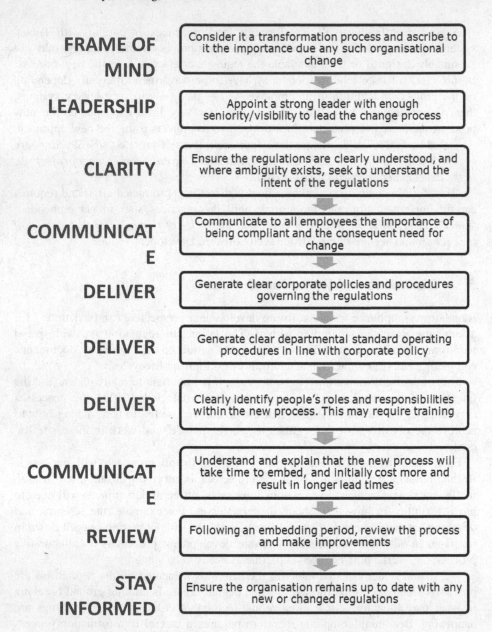

Fig. 3. Suggested steps for regulated process implementation

Acknowledgements. This research is supported by the Science Foundation Ireland (SFI) Stokes Lectureship Programme, grant number 07/SK/I1299, the SFI Principal Investigator Programme, grant number 08/IN.1/I2030 (the funding of this project was awarded by Science Foundation Ireland under a co-funding initiative by the Irish

Government and European Regional Development Fund), and supported in part by Lero - the Irish Software Engineering Research Centre (http://www.lero.ie) grant 10/CE/I1855.

References

1. Anderson, D.J.: Kanban. Blue Hole Press (2010)
2. ANSI/AAMI/IEC. 62304:2006 Medical Device Software-Software life cycle processes. Association for the Advancement of Medical Instrumentation (2006)
3. Basel: Basel II Accord (2004), http://en.wikipedia.org/wiki/Basel_II_Accord (accessed July 31, 2012)
4. Beck, K.: Test Driven Development: By Example. Addison-Wesley Professional (2002)
5. Ben-Menachem, M.: Towards management of software as assets: A literature review with additional sources. Information and Software Technology 50, 241–258 (2008)
6. Boehm, B.: Software Engineering Economics. Prentice Hall (1981)
7. Burn, J.M., Couger, D., Ma, L., Tompkins, H.: Motivating IT professionals-the Hong Kong challenge. In: Proceedings of the Twenty-Fourth Annual Hawaii International Conference on System Sciences, January 8-11, vol. 4, pp. 524–529 (1991)
8. Bush, W.R.: Software, regulation, and domain specificity. Information and Software Technology 49, 44–54 (2007)
9. Campbell, M.K.: Regulations. IEEE Potentials 23, 14–15 (2004)
10. Cawley, O., Richardson, I.: Lessons in Global Software Development – Local to Global Transition within a Regulated Environment. In: European Systems & Software Process Improvement and Innovation, Grenoble, France. Springer (2010)
11. Cawley, O., Richardson, I., Wang, X.: Medical Device Software Development - A Perspective from a Lean Manufacturing Plant. In: O'Connor, R.V., Rout, T., McCaffery, F., Dorling, A. (eds.) SPICE 2011. CCIS, vol. 155, pp. 84–96. Springer, Heidelberg (2011)
12. Cawley, O., Wang, X., Richardson, I.: Lean/Agile Software Development Methodologies in Regulated Environments – State of the Art. In: Abrahamsson, P., Oza, N. (eds.) LESS 2010. LNBIP, vol. 65, pp. 31–36. Springer, Heidelberg (2010)
13. Damian, D.E., Zowghi, D.: The impact of stakeholders' geographical distribution on managing requirements in a multi-site organization. In: Proceedings of the IEEE Joint International Conference on Requirements Engineering, pp. 319–328 (2002)
14. Goldratt, E.M.: The Goal: A Process of Ongoing Improvement. North River Press (1992)
15. Hibbs, C., Jewett, S.C., Sullivan, M.: The Art of Lean Software Development. O'Reilly Media (2009)
16. ISO: ISO 13485:2003 Medical devices – Quality management systems – Requirements for regulatory purposes International Organisation for Standardisation (2003)
17. ISO: ISO 14971:2007 Medical devices – Application of risk management to medical devices. International Organisation for Standardisation (2007)
18. Kettunen, P., Laanti, M.: How to steer an embedded software project: tactics for selecting the software process model. Information and Software Technology 47, 587–608 (2005)
19. Kotter, J.: Leading change: Why Transformation Efforts Fail. Harvard Business Review 73 (1995)
20. Kotter, J.P., Schlesinger, L.A.: Choosing strategies for change. Harvard Business Review 57, 106–114 (1979)

21. Levy, M., Hazzan, O.: Knowledge management in practice: The case of agile software development. In: 2009 ICSE Workshop on Cooperative and Human Aspects on Software Engineering, CHASE 2009, Vancouver, BC, Canada, May 17, pp. 60–65. IEEE Computer Society (2009)
22. Mathiassen, L., Ngwenyama, O.K., Aaen, I.: Managing change in software process improvement. IEEE Software 22, 84–91 (2005)
23. Mcconnell, S.: Problem programmers. IEEE Software 15, 128, 127, 126 (1998)
24. McHugh, M., McCaffery, F., Casey, V.: Standalone Software as an Active Medical Device. In: O'Connor, R.V., Rout, T., McCaffery, F., Dorling, A. (eds.) SPICE 2011. CCIS, vol. 155, pp. 97–107. Springer, Heidelberg (2011)
25. Mullins, L.: Management and Organisational Behaviour. Prentice Hall (2004)
26. Poppendieck, M., Poppendieck, T.: Lean Software Development: An Agile Toolkit. Addison-Wesley Professional (2003)
27. Porter, M.E.: Competitive advantage: creating and sustaining superior performance: with a new introduction. Free Press (1998)
28. Prahalad, C.K., Hamel, G.: The Core Competence of the Corporation. Harvard Business Review 68, 79–91 (1990)
29. OECD: Untangling intangible assets. OECD Observer, 13–15 (2011)
30. Rasmussen, R., Hughes, T., Jenks, J.R., Skach, J.: Adopting Agile in an FDA Regulated Environment. In: Agile Conference (2009)
31. Roberts Jr., T.L., Gibson, M.L., Fields, K.T., Rainer Jr., R.K.: Factors that impact implementing a system development methodology. IEEE Transactions on Software Engineering 24, 640–649 (1998)
32. Robillard, P.N.: The role of knowledge in software development. Commun. ACM 42, 87–92 (1999)
33. Rottier, P.A., Rodrigues, V.: Agile Development in a Medical Device Company. In: AGILE 2008 Conference (2008)
34. Sharp, H., Hall, T.: An initial investigation of software practitioners' motivation. In: Proceedings of the 2009 ICSE Workshop on Cooperative and Human Aspects on Software Engineering. IEEE Computer Society (2009)
35. Small, A.W., Downey, E.A.: Managing change: some important aspects. In: Proceedings of the Change Management and the New Industrial Revolution, IEMC 2001, pp. 50–57 (2001)
36. SOX: Sarbanes-Oxley Act of 2002 (2002), http://www.sec.gov/about/laws.shtml#sox2002 (accessed July 31, 2012)
37. THE-FREE-DICTIONARY 2011. Regulations
38. Treude, C., Barzilay, O., Storey, M.-A.: How do programmers ask and answer questions on the web (NIER track). In: Proceedings of the 33rd International Conference on Software Engineering, Waikiki, Honolulu, HI, USA. ACM (2011)
39. Vogel, D.A.: Medical Device Software Verification, Validation and Compliance. Artech House Publishers (2010)
40. Ye, Y., Nakakoji, K., Yamamoto, Y.: The economy of collective attention for situated knowledge collaboration in software development. In: Proceedings of the 2008 International Workshop on Cooperative and Human Aspects of Software Engineering, Leipzig, Germany. ACM (2008)
41. Ziegler, A.S.: Regulation. Annals of the New York Academy of Sciences 1093, 339–349 (2006)

An Architecture and Reference Implementation of an Open Health Information Mediator: Enabling Interoperability in the Rwandan Health Information Exchange

Ryan Crichton[1,2], Deshendran Moodley[1], Anban Pillay[1], Richard Gakuba[3], and Christopher J. Seebregts[1,2,4]

[1] Health Architecture Laboratory, Centre for Artificial Intelligence Research, University of KwaZulu-Natal and Council for Scientific and Industrial Research, Durban, South Africa
[2] Jembi Health Systems, Cape Town and Durban, South Africa
[3] eHealth Coordination Unit, Ministry of Health, Rwanda
[4] Medical Research Council, Cape Town, South Africa

Abstract. Rwanda, one of the smallest and most densely populated countries in Africa, has made rapid and substantial progress towards designing and deploying a national health information system. One of the more challenging aspects of the system is the design of an architecture to support: interoperability between existing health information systems already in use in the country; incremental extension into a fully integrated national health information system without substantial re-engineering; and scaling, from a single district in the initial phase, to national level without requiring a fundamental change in technology or design paradigm. This paper describes the key requirements and the design of the current architecture using the ISO/IEC/IEEE 42010 standard architecture descriptions. The architecture takes an Enterprise Service Bus approach. A partial implementation and preliminary analysis of the architecture is given. Since these challenges are experienced by other developing African countries, the next steps involves creating a generic architecture that can be reused for health information exchange in other developing African countries.

Keywords: interoperability, national health information system architecture, enterprise service bus, health information exchange.

1 Introduction

The current landscape of health information systems, especially in the developing world, is mostly characterised by fragmented, piecemeal applications deployed by multiple organizations [1,4]. Applications are usually custom built to satisfy very specific needs, using different architectures and technologies, with interoperability low on the list of priorities. While these systems may be useful in a specific domain, their integration into a coherent national health information

J. Weber and I. Perseil (Eds.): FHIES 2012, LNCS 7789, pp. 87–104, 2013.

system (NHIS) is challenging. One potential solution to enable interoperability is to implement a mediator component that facilitates information exchange and orchestration between participating health information systems and applications in the NHIS, including point of service applications and shared registries and services.

In our previous work [21] we identified general challenges and requirements for designing and developing NHIS architectures in developing African countries. In this paper we identify specific interoperability challenges and requirements for the Rwandan NHIS and describe the design and implementation of an Health Information Mediator (HIM) that has been adopted in Rwanda for use in its NHIS. In section 2 we describe the background to the Rwandan NHIS. Section 3 provides the key requirements and challenges for interoperability that informed the design of the HIM. The architecture of the HIM is presented in section 4 and section 5 gives an analysis of this architecture. In section 6 the implementation of the architecture is briefly described and we draw our conclusions in section 7.

2 Background: A National Health Information System for Rwanda

The Rwanda Ministry of Health (MoH) has already made significant progress in developing a country-level NHIS, that includes, among others, community health systems, health management information systems and the national roll-out of an electronic medical record application [20]. The Rwanda Health Enterprise Architecture (RHEA) project, led by the Rwanda MoH and supported by a consortium of partners and donors has developed an Health Information Exchange to facilitate interoperability between individual health information systems and applications. We follow Dixon et al [8] and define a health information exchange (HIE) broadly as "the sharing of clinical and administrative healthcare data among healthcare institutions, providers, and data repositories."

Implementation of the Rwandan HIE will be achieved in several phases. The first phase will implement foundational components, including client, professionals and facilities registries, a terminology service and a shared health record, to improve interoperability between two point of care information systems supporting maternal health in the Rwamagana district, including 15 health centers. The two point of care systems being implemented and maintained by the Rwandan MoH are implementations of OpenMRS [18,2,26], an Electronic Medial Record (EMR) system and RapidSMS, an SMS based data collection tool that is currently being used by community health workers. RapidSMS allows community health workers (CHWs) in Rwanda to submit maternal and child health information to a central server using SMS based messages from mobile phones. There are many CHWs within Rwanda and this information plays an important role in monitoring the progress of pregnant women and the health of children where frequent visits to clinics are not possible. In subsequent phases, the HIE will need to accommodate other applications and use cases and also scale, nationally.

The HIE's main function is to enable the point of care systems currently implemented in Rwanda to connect and inter-operate more easily. Using the HIE, the MoH plans to promote data re-use between the connected systems and to facilitate information sharing. It also aims to provide patients with a continuity of care record [11] to enable access to a patient's clinical information from different health facilities thus improving the tracking of patients and reducing the number of patients lost-to-follow-up.

The first phase involves deploying a set of foundational infrastructure services that provide services to point of care applications, initially, OpenMRS and RapidSMS. The HIE will allow the systems to share clinical information and ensure that shared information uniquely identifies the patient, provider and facility within the information exchange (Figure 1).

The foundational infrastructure services are:

- Shared Health Record
  - This system persists and responds to queries for an appropriate subset of the patient's longitudinal, patient-centric medical record.
- Client Registry
  - This system persists and responds to queries for a patient's demographic and identifying information used to uniquely identify patients.
- Facility Registry
  - This system persists and responds to queries for data of the facilities participating in the information exchange. This is primarily used to maintain current and valid facility codes required in transactions.
- Professional Registry
  - This system persists and responds to queries for information about health care professionals who work at participating health care facilities in the information exchange. This is primarily used to uniquely identify health care professionals within the HIE.
- Terminology Service
  - This system stores all the clinical code systems (eg. LOINC, ICD10 and country specific code systems) that will be used within the HIE and facilitates verification and mapping between codes. It exposes endpoints that allow codes to be verified against the stored code systems.

3   Interoperability: Challenges and Requirements

The interoperability layer, shown in figure 1, is the cornerstone of the Rwandan HIE architecture and its design has significant impact on the effectiveness, scalability, sustainability and adaptability of the overall system. In the sections that follow we enumerate the challenges and requirements, suggest and explain a possible design of an architecture for this interoperability layer and give a preliminary analysis of it effectiveness when applied to the Rwandan HIE.

The design was informed by the following requirements and challenges that were identified from studying the situation in Rwandan and with knowledge of how health informations systems are deployed in low resource settings:

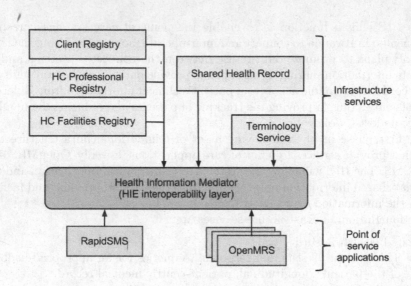

Fig. 1. The architecture of the Rwandan Health Information Exchange

Facilitate Interoperability between Disparate and Heterogeneous Systems, Both Existing and Future

In the context of the Rwandan NHIS, the HIE initially allows the OpenMRS and RapidSMS systems to inter-operate with the infrastructure services (client registry, provider registry, facility registry and the shared health record) in order to share information. Each system embodies a different technology and architecture and the interoperability layer enables these systems to interact effectively.

The interoperability layer must provide mechanisms to allow existing disparate and heterogeneous systems to be incorporated into the HIE with minimal changes to the systems and still allow for local autonomy. The systems need to be able to grow and develop independently of the overall HIE and the other systems participating in the HIE. The architecture must be technology agnostic, with minimal restrictions on the technologies used within participating systems. Challenges include syntactic, semantic and process or pragmatic heterogeneity [22,14].

Adapt and Scale within a Changing Environment

The focus of the current project is to enable the sharing of maternal health information between point of service applications in a single district. However, this architecture will also need to adapt to new requirements and grow as the project progresses. It has to be designed to expand such that the services may be readily expanded to other districts in Rwanda, to incorporate additional domains of health care (for example, the HIV/TB programmes) and allow other systems to be incorporated as part of the growth of the HIE.

The architecture must support incremental development and evolution of the HIE and also must be able to grow as the country's needs expand over time. This is especially true in low-resource environments where many organizations implement disparate information systems for a variety of purposes [3]. An essential feature of a HIE is its ability to cope with change. The architecture must be flexible enough to deal with changing and evolving NHIS requirements.

The system must also be able to scale, in terms of transaction volume, geographical locations and increased functionality.

Local Changes Should Not Propagate through the System

In Rwanda, development teams in different organizations design and maintain participating systems such as OpenMRS, RapidSMS and the infrastructure services. Currently, there are 14 partners working on the Rwandan HIE with 7 different development teams working on the various participating systems that must be able to develop independently without affecting other systems. Participating systems will need to balance local requirements and NHIS requirements, but from a practical perspective development teams will often prioritise local requirements. Changes to participating systems should have minimal effect on other systems and systems must also be protected as much as possible from changes to infrastructure services. All systems must still maintain a large degree of local autonomy, especially since these systems are implemented and maintained by a variety of disparate organizations.

Provide a Low Barrier to Entry to Connect New and Legacy Systems

Implementing partners have development teams distributed around the world with varying degrees of expertise and technical skills. Inter-operating with the infrastructure services must be simple and require minimal effort both for current as well as new technical teams. A number of existing health information systems including the OpenMRS implementations and the RapidSMS implementation existed before the HIE was conceived.

The HIE should reduce the burden of connecting new and legacy systems participating in the HIE. The approach toward integration of legacy systems should be to 'embrace and extend' and not to 'rip and replace'. The architecture must provide a minimal barrier to entry to incorporate a system into the HIE and reduce the overhead required to modify a particular system to participate in the HIE. This feature will maximize the existing investment in legacy applications and help prevent useful and functioning legacy applications from being abandoned unnecessarily.

4   Architecture of the Health Information Mediator

In order to overcome the challenges and fulfill the requirements for interoperability identified in section 3, we introduce a new component, the Health Information

Mediator (HIM) (figure 2). The design and implementation of the HIM draws heavily from two technologies that were evaluated in the initial stages of the Rwandan project. The first, Mirth Connect (Mirth Corporation), is an open integration engine for health information systems. However, the Rwandan project required complex orchestrations that Mirth Connect could not easily support and it was simpler to directly use the underlying Mule ESB [16] platform on which Mirth Connect is built to perform orchestration. We also reviewed and setup the reference implementation of the Canada Health Infoway (CHI) EHR Blueprint [7,19]. In the CHI HIE implementation the interoperability and orchestration functions are provided by Biztalk (Microsoft Corporation), supplemented by Everest, an HL7[1] version 3 adapter and open C# library. However, Biztalk is expensive to license and maintain and HL7 version 3 is a difficult messaging specification to implement in low resource settings due to its complexity and verbose nature.

In this section, we describe the architecture of the HIM using ISO 42010 architecture descriptions [17,10]. ISO/IEC FDIS 42010 provides a formal language and a metamodel for creating, analysing and sustaining architecture descriptions. An architecture can be described by a number of architectural views with each view framing a number of concerns (including requirements) of different groups of stakeholders with an interest in the system. Together, these views make up the architecture description. Based on the requirements identified in section 3, three major views of the HIM architecture and their associated concerns are described below.

4.1   Logical View

This view describes the overall functionality of the system. The model kinds include custom diagrams showing how transactions flow through the architecture. It frames the following concerns:

- The architecture must facilitate interoperability between heterogeneous systems
- The architecture must provide a low barrier to entry to connect both new and legacy systems
- Changes should be kept local and not propagate through the system

Based on these requirements, we have designed the HIM as a middleware system to enable interoperability between participating systems and infrastructure services. The HIM is based on the Enterprise Service Bus (ESB) architectural model.

An ESB [5,25] is a middleware system that facilitates interoperability by providing a central bus that manages all communications between participating systems. Since the components within an ESB are loosely coupled and can run completely independently of each other, each component can still function independently when other components fail.

---

[1] HL7 is a standard messaging format for data within the health domain.

ESB is a well established architectural model for meeting the requirements associated with interoperability between distributed and disparate systems that has previously been applied to the problem of interoperability between disparate health information systems [24,15].

All participating systems in the HIE are represented as services. Systems that provide services to other systems are termed service providers, while systems that make requests of other systems are termed service requesters. All service requests are made via the HIM. The HIM thus provides mediation and orchestration functions within the system.

Our approach contains three major components described by the following 3-tuple:

$$HIM = \{I, P, M\}$$

where HIM is the Health Information Mediator, I is the Interface component, P is the Persistence component and M is the Mediation component.

Figure 2 shows the order in which transactions flow through each of the components.

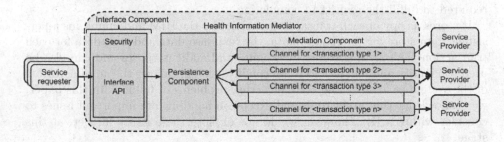

Fig. 2. Overview of components in the HIM architecture

Each of these components are described below:

I - Interface Component. All interactions are carried out via the HIM. The interface component exposes an application programming interface (API) that allows systems or applications to make service requests through the HIE. It is responsible for defining and handling all incoming service requests. Service requests are received using a standard protocol (e.g. HTTP) and translated into a common internal format that is accessible by the other components in the layer (e.g. Java Objects). The request is then passed to the persistence component for further processing.

This component not only provides a single and consistent entry point for all service requests, but also enforces security and access policies for the HIE.

A single point of access simplifies interactions with the HIE as the systems can make service requests without needing to know the location or security requirements of the service providers.

The API currently uses web services which affords the HIM greater flexibility when connecting systems using varying platforms and technologies. The functions provided by the API are defined according to the requirements of the HIE implementation. In the Rwandan use case this includes functions to save and query a patient's clinical record within the shared health record and to query and update records in the client, provider and facility registries.

This component also provides a central place for defining and applying advanced security policies. In this component, access to the API and access to specific functions of the API should be strictly controlled. The component also allows data-level security policies to be applied, if needed. In this paper, we have not addressed the complexities of defining how these security policies could be applied in order to focus on the architectural significance of security and not the implementation details.

P - Persistence Component. This component receives authorised service requests from the interface component and starts and monitors a transaction required to fulfill the request to completion.

It stores a copy of each transaction received by the HIM and maintains a persistent data store for the request data, the response data and metadata for each transaction. This data is stored for logging and audit purposes and can also be used to identify and handle exception conditions. This allows the administrators of the system to identify and solve recurring problems or failures. In this paper, we acknowledge that audit trails and exception handling are important issues to consider within a HIE, however we do not explore these issues further, at this stage.

Transaction metadata allow administrators of the system to monitor transactions and gauge the health of the system. This is useful for discovering bottlenecks and performance problems.

M - Mediation Component. The mediation component executes transactions. Its main functions are orchestration and message translation.

The mediation component is made up of a number of transaction channels. A channel is provided for each transaction type, e.g. a transaction type to save a patient's encounter. It contains the necessary logic to normalise, orchestrate and de-normalise that transaction. Each function exposed by the API in the interface component maps to a transaction type and therefore to a transaction channel.

Below we describe the process that occurs within a single transaction channel contained within the mediation component.

Figure 3 shows the inner workings of the transaction mediation component described earlier. Each transaction type has its own transaction channel. The diagram represents the workflow within a single transaction channel.

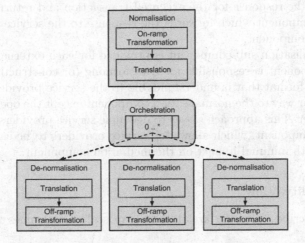

Fig. 3. The workflow of a transaction channel within the transaction mediation component

A transaction channel always begins with a normalisation sub-component. This sub-component transforms the request message contained within a transaction to a normalised state. After this process the transaction data must be in a consistent and predictable format to allow components following this to process it in a predictable fashion, no matter what format it arrived in. This process consists of 2 operations. Firstly, an on-ramp transformation is applied. This ensures syntactic interoperability for the transaction. For example, if the transaction arrives from a legacy application that only supported exporting data in a custom XML format, this process would ensure that the XML is transformed into a form that the rest of the exchange can understand, e.g. an HL7 version 2 message. Secondly, a translation operation is invoked. This operation is responsible for ensuring the codes and code systems used within the transaction are translated to a standard set of vocabulary or clinical terms that have a common interpretation by other components of the HIM. This involves a call to the terminology service to translate and verify that the codes used within the transaction are in or are translated to an internal standard vocabulary. The terminology server is responsible for maintaining a standard vocabulary and mappings to other vocabularies used by participating systems. In this way semantic interoperability between service requesters and providers is achieved.

Following this, the transaction is sent to the orchestration sub-component. This sub-component is responsible for performing implementation-specific orchestration for the current transaction. The process of orchestration is described in Peltz et al [23]. The aim of the orchestration component is to execute the received transaction and perform any consequent action(s) required for this transaction. This could include 0 or more calls to external services. This component also compiles the response for the executed transaction and returns this to the persistence component which forwards the response to the service requester via the interface component.

A de-normalisation sub-component is provided for each external service call. This sub-component is responsible for transforming (or constructing) a service request into a format that is understandable to the service provider. This operates in a similar way to the normalisation component except the operations occur in reverse order. This approach serves to decouple service providers from the orchestration component, which allows for service providers to be easily modified or replaced with minimal impact on the mediation component.

4.2   Scalability View

This view describes how the architecture can scale and frames the following concern:

– The architecture must scale in terms of the number and volume of transactions

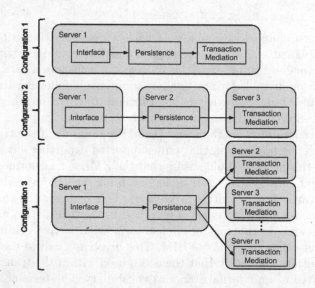

Fig. 4. Scalability configurations of the HIM architecture

Figure 4 show the scalability of the architecture. In the architecture there are 3 major components; the interface API, the persistence component and the mediation component. Each of these components are loosely coupled to allow them to be deployed across different servers. This is shown in 'Configuration 2' in figure 4. The 3 components are responsible for separate units of work. This loose coupling allows the components to be spread over different hardware as long as they can communicate over a network. The ESB architectural model used for this architecture ensures that the components are loosely coupled and can be deployed distributedly.

It is also feasible to further separate the persistence component and the transaction mediation component through clustering. The persistence component performs the static function of persisting any transaction that passes through it. As this function is not dynamic it could easily be replicated over multiple servers with the provision that the data store is kept in sync. This component could also be invoked in an asynchronous fashion as the mediation component subsequent to it does not require this process to complete in order to continue.

The transaction mediation component can be scaled horizontally. The transaction mediation component holds a set of channels, one for each transaction type that is supported by the implementation. Each of these channels encapsulates information about how each transaction should be transformed and orchestrated. Each transaction channel runs independently which allows for deployment of the channels across different servers. This is shown in configuration 3 in figure 4.

These configurations show two important aspects of the architecture. Firstly performance in terms of volumes of transactions, i.e. splitting the load between different servers increases the capability of the system to handle and process a higher volume of transactions timeously. Additional servers can be introduced as transaction volumes grow . Secondly, robustness. Since each of the three components are responsible for separate units of work and individual components can be replicated over different physical machines to provide redundancy. The number of instances of each component can be varied depending on the transaction types and processing requirements.

4.3   Adaptability View

This view shows the architecture's ability to grow with a country's NHIS and how new services can be easily added or changed within the architecture.

This view frames the following concern:

– The architecture must be adaptable in a changing environment

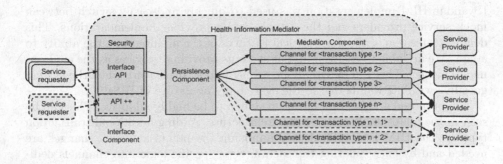

Fig. 5. Adaptability of the HIM architecture

Adaptability is an important consideration for this architecture. Figure 5 shows how additional services could be added to the architecture. As can be seen, to add additional services the interface component's API needs to be extended to add new API endpoints for each new function that needs to be supported. The persistence component is generic enough that it does not require any change to process new types of service requests. The transaction mediation component is where most of the changes are required. This component is designed to encapsulate transaction mediation logic for each transaction type. A new transaction channel can easily be added along side the others to support a new type of service request. The channel will encapsulate all the logic for normalising the transaction, executing the necessary orchestration steps and to de-normalise the transaction when an external service orchestration call is made. This encapsulation simplifies the addition of new service request types as functionality increases and the HIE expands.

5   Analysis

In this section the HIM architecture is analysed against the requirements set out in section 3. This HIM architecture is currently being used to drive the development of the Rwandan HIE. The implementation and deployment of the first phase of the HIE in Rwanda is currently underway and the architecture is already showing benefit during this process. The discussion below is based on our experiences of implementing this architecture.

One of the core requirements of the HIE is to allow disparate systems to connect to each other easily. These could be legacy or new systems built by various international or local organizations. The architecture accomplishes this by enforcing a single interface API to connect to the HIE. This API hides the complexity of the HIE as well as the underlying system(s) that are invoked to fulfill service requests. This architecture also protects the applications requesting services from changes that will inevitably occur to service providers, their API's or as a result of migration to a different location. This enables and supports local autonomy of the participating systems.

As new services are being developed and deployed for the Rwandan NHIS the Rwandan HIM implementation was used to quickly and easily switch between mock service providers and the actual service provider implementations. This demonstrates one of the most critical features of the architecture; the ability to adapt. We are able to easily swap-out systems providing services as the environment changes. This will inevitably be a very important feature when the system goes live within Rwanda due to the ever changing nature of HISs.

The proposed architecture has been shown to be highly adaptive. This can be seen in the adaptability view of the architecture. Adding additional transaction types to the HIM is simplified by minimising the points at which changes are needed and by encapsulating transaction type specific logic into channels dedicated to specific transactions. This allows the architecture to adapt effectively as the HIE environment and functionality grows.

One of the major benefits of this architecture is that is does not prescribe the use of a particular data exchange format. There are many messaging standards available in the health domain for syntactic interoperability, each with different structures for representing data. Standards exist for various types of messaging needs. For example, sending clinical information (HL7 v2, HL7 v3, OpenEHR Archetypes [6,13,9]) or aggregate health information for reporting (SDMX-HD [3]). A defacto standard for health care messaging has yet to emerge [9]. New standards will emerge over time and current standards will fall away. Given these facts we can see that no single standard will ever be sufficient for all messaging needs. Therefore, the architecture must support current and future standards for syntactic interoperability. In the proposed architecture any data can be exchanged as long as we have normalisation and de-normalisation transforms defined to allow the data format to be transformed into and out of a form that the mediation component can understand and orchestrate. This affords the architecture greater flexibility in the types of data that can flow through it and allows the architecture to cater for multiple domains of health care even if the standard data exchange formats used within those domains are very different. This approach also future proofs the architecture against the inevitable change and evolution that will occur in the syntactic interoperability domain in health care.

A criticism of the architecture presented here is that it does not draw a clear line between parts of the system that are implementation specific and parts that can be part of a more general interoperability framework. Within the interface component and the mediation component there are parts that need to be defined depending on the API and business processes that are being implemented. These parts are implementation specific. The interface component defines an API that will be heavily driven by implementation needs and the mediation component defines orchestrations that are defined by the implementation as well as on-ramp steps and off-ramp steps that would depend on the data representations used within that implementation. It would be beneficial to identify the implementation specific aspects of this architecture so that a general interoperability framework can be extracted and implementation specific configuration can be plugged-in as needed. The current architecture does not account for this. This can be explored in future work.

The security architecture is also not expanded upon greatly in this architecture. It is identified that having a common entry point into the HIM is beneficial in this regard as there is only a single endpoint to secure, however there are much greater considerations that need to be identified. Two main examples are: restricting transactions that specific applications can execute within the interoperability layer and providing data level security on the clinical information that passes through the system.

The HIM architecture was conceived by studying the challenges and requirements of NHISs in a low resource setting. These challenges led us to an architecture that relies on a central component (the HIM) that co-ordinates all the interaction within the HIE. This design choice has its benefits as well as its challenges. Having a central component gives the benefit of easing the burden of implementing interoperability between HISs as the infrastructure only need to be deployed once and the HIM can simplify the burden of connecting to a HIE. It also gives a country central control over the transactions supported within the HIE. Having a central component that is responsible for orchestration of all the transactions also allows the client systems to be so-called 'dumb clients' and only interact with the system in a simple manner. This enables quicker and easier integration that will help resource constrained projects to connect their systems to the HIE. The design also keeps much of the communication between systems in the datacentre where communication is quick and responsive. Client systems in low resource setting are often on slow networks that are often unresponsive or out of order. Minimal communication with a single central component allows clients to communicate effectively with the little bandwidth that they have. On the other hand, having a central component also has certain negative aspects. A central component that the entire HIE relies on introduces a single point of failure. Also, if any changes need to be make to the transactions that the HIE supports the central component need to be changed and all other systems have to wait until these changes are implemented before they can utilise the new transactions. The HIM would likely be controlled by a government entity and the client systems are often controlled by a wide variety of organizations that can move much more quickly than a government entity. Thus, problems could be encountered if the government entity is not responsive enough to change requests.

Alternative design approaches could do away with a central component and expect the client to know how to communicate among themselves ('smart clients' or service choreography). In our case the central approach seemed most appropriate due to the fact that we are working in a low resource setting. The benefits for a low resource setting out-weighed the negatives listed above, however, the authors note that this will not always be the case in other settings.

Overall, the architecture fulfills the key requirements needed to implement a HIE interoperability architecture for a NHIS in Rwanda. This has been proven to work in a lab environment as the implementation for the Rwandan HIE is being developed as well as in production as the Rwandan HIE begins to be rolled out. Many of these requirements are not specific to Rwanda and can be applied to other low-resource settings where a HIE is needed. Therefore, the authors believe this architecture is highly applicable for use in other countries.

6   Implementation and Future Work

The HIM architecture, described above was implemented and successfully deployed with the other HIE components in Rwanda during September 2012. The current system connects two health facilities in the Rwamagana district to the HIE deployed in the national datacentre in Kigali[2].

---

[2] See the implementation blog at
   http://rwandahie.blogspot.com/2012/09/click.html

The Infrastructure services that form the rest of the Rwandan HIE were implemented by different parties utilising a wide variety of open source projects, which are listed below:

- Shared Health Record: OpenMRS (OpenMRS Foundation, Regenstrief Institute and Partners in Health)
- Client Registry: OpenEMPI (SYSNET International)
- Provider Registry: a custom open source webapp built on OpenLDAP (Intrahealth)
- Facility Registry: ResourceMapper (InSTEDD)
- Terminology service: Apelon DTS (Apelon Inc.) and a webapp frontend (Jembi Health Systems NPC).

The Rwandan HIM was developed on the open source Mule ESB [16] platform, and incorporates a RESTful web services approach [12]. The implementation and field experience sets the foundation towards creating an Open Health Information Mediator (OpenHIM). The architecture as well as the implemented components of the Rwandan HIM are general enough to allow their re-use in other settings. The aim is to release the Rwandan HIM as open source and for it to serve as the reference implementation for the OpenHIM. The next step is to establish an open community around OpenHIM to provide participation from other stakeholders and to promote its adoption and to facilitate the creation of Health Information Exchanges in other low resource settings.

7   Conclusion

In this paper we have identified the need for an interoperability architecture to solve the problem of interoperability between many disparate health information systems. The Rwandan HIE use case was used to drive the identification of the requirements for this middleware layer, however, these requirements are largely applicable to other contexts. We introduce the HIM architecture that attempts to solve the problems identified by the requirements. ISO 42010 is utilised to describe this architecture so that we can ensure all of the concerns are satisfied by utilising 3 different views of the architecture.

The HIM architecture description presents a proposed solution for interoperability architectures for use in low-resource countries like Rwanda and attempts to formalise the description of such an architecture so that it can be reused in other settings. The architecture is analysed using experience in implementing the architecture for use in the Rwandan HIE. It is identified that the architecture solves the problems identified by the requirements, however, it fails to provide a clear separation between the implementation specific configuration and the framework for a more general architecture. Overall, the architecture provides a solution to the major problems faced when attempting to facilitate interoperability between many disparate health information systems and it has proven in practice to be an appropriate, adaptable and scalable solution.

Acknowledgements. The authors wish to acknowledge the support of the Rwanda Ministry of Health and, in particular, Gilbert Uwayezo and Daniel Murenzi who with the National eHealth Coordinator, Dr Richard Gakuba, manage the national rollout of health IT as well as advisers, Elizabeth Peloso and Randy Wilson. Significant inputs were received from the Rwanda Health Enterprise Architecture (RHEA) and Rwanda Health Information Exchange (RHIE) project teams, including Wayne Naidoo, Carl Fourie, Hannes Venter, Mead Walker, Beatriz de Faria Leao, Paul Biondich, Shaun Grannis, Eduardo Jezierski, Dykki Settle, Odysseas Pentakalos and Bob Joliffe. Additional support was obtained from Mohawk College in Canada (in particular, Derek Ritz, Ted Scott, Justin Fyfe and Duane Bender) and eZ-Vida in Brazil (in particular, Dr Lincoln Moura and Ricardo Quintano Neira).

The RHEA project is funded by grants from the IDRC (Open Architectures, Standards and Information Systems (OASIS II) - Developing Capacity, Sharing Knowledge and Good Principles Across eHealth in Africa. Grant Number: 105708), the Rockefeller Foundation (Open eHealth Enterprise Architecture Framework and Strategy Development for the Global South; Grant Number: 2009 THS 328) and the Health Informatics Public Private Partnership Project funded by the President's Emergency Plan for AIDS Relief (PEPFAR). This research has been supported by funding from the President's Emergency Plan for AIDS Relief (PEPFAR) through a CDC cooperative agreement with Cardno Emerging Markets, Cooperative Agreement #PS002068. The HEAL project is funded by grants from the Rockefeller Foundation (Establishing a Health Enterprise Architecture Lab, a research laboratory focused on the application of enterprise architecture and health informatics to low-resource settings, Grant Number: 2010 THS 347) and the IDRC (Health Enterprise Architecture Laboratory (HEAL), Grant Number: 106452-001). The REACH (Research in Enterprise Architecture for Coordinating Healthcare) project was also funded by the IDRC through ecGroup (Derek Ritz).

References

1. AbouZahr, C., Boerma, T.: Health information systems: the foundations of public health. Bulletin of the World Health Organization 83(8), 578–583 (2005)
2. Allen, C., Jazayeri, D., Miranda, J., Biondich, P.G., Mamlin, B.W., Wolfe, B.A., Seebregts, C., Lesh, N., Tierney, W.M., Fraser, H.S.: Experience in implementing the OpenMRS medical record system to support HIV treatment in Rwanda. Studies in Health Technology and Informatics 129(pt. 1), 382–386 (2007)
3. Braa, J., Kanter, A.S., Lesh, N., Crichton, R., Jolliffe, B., Sæbø, J., Kossi, E., Seebregts, C.J.: Comprehensive yet scalable health information systems for low resource settings: a collaborative effort in Sierra Leone. In: AMIA Annual Symposium Proceedings, vol. 2010, pp. 372–376 (2010)
4. Braa, J., Muquinge, H.: Building collaborative networks in Africa on health information systems and open source software development - Experience from the HISP/BEANISH network. IST Africa (2007)

5. Chappell, D.: Enterprise Service Bus: Theory in Practice. O'Reilly Media (July 2004)
6. Chen, R.: Towards interoperable and knowledge-based electronic health records using archetype methodology. PhD thesis, Department of Biomedical Engineering, Linköpings universitet (2009)
7. CHI: EHRS Blueprint. An Interoperable EHR Framework. Executive Overview
8. Dixon, B.E., Zafar, A., Marc Overhage, J.: A framework for evaluating the costs, effort, and value of nationwide health information exchange. JAMIA 17(3), 295–301 (2010)
9. Eichelberg, M., Aden, T., Riesmeier, J., Dogac, A., Laleci, G.B.: A survey and analysis of Electronic Healthcare Record standards. ACM Comput. Surv. 37(4), 277–315 (2005)
10. Emery, D., Hilliard, R.: Updating IEEE 1471: Architecture Frameworks and Other Topics. In: Seventh Working IEEE/IFIP Conference on Software Architecture (WICSA 2008), pp. 303–306. IEEE, Washington, DC (2008)
11. Ferranti, J.M., Musser, R.C., Kawamoto, K., Hammond, W.E.: The Clinical Document Architecture and the Continuity of Care Record: A Critical Analysis. Journal of the American Medical Informatics Association 13(3), 245–252 (2006)
12. Fielding, R.T.: Architectural styles and the design of network-based software architectures. PhD thesis, University of California, Irvine, CA, USA (2000)
13. Garde, S., Chen, R., Leslie, H., Beale, T., McNicoll, I., Heard, S.: Archetype-Based Knowledge Management for Semantic Interoperability of Electronic Health Records, pp. 1007–1011. IOS Press (2009)
14. Gibbons, P., Arzt, N., Burke-Beebe, S., Chute, C., Dickinson, G., Flewelling, T., Jepsen, T., Kamens, D., Larson, J., Ritter, J., Rozen, M., Selover, S., Stanford, J.: Coming to Terms: Scoping Interoperability for Health Care. Technical report, Health Level Seven EHR Interoperability Work Group (February 2007)
15. IBM: IBM Enterprise Service Bus for Healthcare. Technical report (2010)
16. MuleSoft Inc.: What is Mule ESB? (2012), http://www.mulesoft.org/what-mule-esb
17. ISO: ISO/IEC FDIS 42010 IEEE P42010/D9. Systems and software engineering - Architecture description. Technical report, ISO (March 2011)
18. Mamlin, B.W., Biondich, P.G., Wolfe, B.A., Fraser, H., Jazayeri, D., Allen, C., Miranda, J., Tierney, W.M.: Cooking up an open source EMR for developing countries: OpenMRS - a recipe for successful collaboration. In: AMIA Symposium, pp. 529–533 (2006)
19. Duane, B., Yendt, M., Minaji, B.: Developing an Open Source Reference Implementation of the Canadian Electronic Health Records Solution. Open Source Business Resource, Health and Life Sciences (November 2008)
20. Ministry of Health, Rwanda: Health Sector Strategic Plan (July 2009-June 2012)
21. Moodley, D., Pillay, A.W., Seebregts, C.J.: Position Paper: Researching and Developing Open Architectures for National Health Information Systems in Developing African Countries. In: Liu, Z., Wassyng, A. (eds.) FHIES 2011. LNCS, vol. 7151, pp. 129–139. Springer, Heidelberg (2012)
22. Ouksel, A.M., Sheth, A.: Semantic interoperability in global information systems. SIGMOD Rec. 28(1), 5–12 (1999)
23. Peltz, C.: Web services orchestration and choreography. Computer 36(10), 46–52 (2003)

24. Ryan, A., Eklund, P.: The Health Service Bus: an architecture and case study in achieving interoperability in healthcare. Studies in Health Technology and Informatics 160(pt. 2), 922–926 (2010)
25. Schmidt, M.T., Hutchison, B., Lambros, P., Phippen, R.: The Enterprise Service Bus: Making service-oriented architecture real. IBM Systems Journal 44(4), 781–797 (2005)
26. Seebregts, C.J., Mamlin, B.W., Biondich, P.G., Fraser, H.S.F., Wolfe, B.A., Jazayeri, D., Allen, C., Miranda, J., Baker, E., Musinguzi, N., Kayiwa, D., Fourie, C., Lesh, N., Kanter, A., Yiannoutsos, C.T., Bailey, C.: The OpenMRS Implementers Network. International Journal of Medical Informatics 78(11), 711–720 (2009)

O_{wl}O_{nt}DB: A Scalable Reasoning System for OWL 2 RL Ontologies with Large ABoxes

Rokan Uddin Faruqui and Wendy MacCaull

Centre for Logic and Information
St. Francis Xavier University
Nova Scotia, Canada
{x2010mcd,wmaccaul}@stfx.ca

Abstract. Ontologies are becoming increasingly important in large-scale information systems such as healthcare systems. Ontologies can represent knowledge from clinical guidelines, standards, and practices used in the healthcare sector and may be used to drive decision support systems for healthcare, as well as store data (facts) about patients. Real-life ontologies may get very large (with millions of facts or instances). The effective use of ontologies requires not only a well-designed and well-defined ontology language, but also adequate support from reasoning tools. Main memory-based reasoners are not suitable for reasoning over large ontologies due to the high time and space complexity of their reasoning algorithms. In this paper, we present OwlOntDB, a scalable reasoning system for OWL 2 RL ontologies with a large number of instances, i.e., large ABoxes. We use a logic-based approach to develop the reasoning system by extending the Description Logic Programs (DLP) mapping between OWL 1 ontologies and datalog rules, to accommodate the new features of OWL 2 RL. We first use a standard DL reasoner to create a complete class hierarchy from an OWL 2 RL ontology, and translate each axiom and fact from the ontology to its equivalent datalog rule(s) using the extended DLP mapping. We materialize the ontology to infer implicit knowledge using a novel database-driven forward chaining method, storing asserted and inferred knowledge in a relational database. We evaluate queries using a modified SPARQL-DL API over the relational database. We show our system performs favourably with respect to query evaluation when compared to two main-memory based reasoners on several ontologies with large datasets including a healthcare ontology.

Keywords: Ontology, Knowledge Representation, Healthcare System, Scalable Reasoner, OWL 2 RL.

1 Introduction

Ontologies are becoming increasingly important in large-scale information systems such as healthcare systems. Ontologies can represent knowledge from clinical guidelines, standards, and practices used in the healthcare sector and may be used to drive decision support systems for healthcare. Applications for these types of systems use large ontologies, i.e., ontologies with a large number

J. Weber and I. Perseil (Eds.): FHIES 2012, LNCS 7789, pp. 105–123, 2013.
© Springer-Verlag Berlin Heidelberg 2013

(millions) of instances. The W3C recommends the use of the Web Ontology Language (OWL), a semantic markup language, which provides a formal syntax and semantics to represent ontologies and paves the way for manipulating ontologies effectively [20]. However, the effective use of ontologies requires not only a well-designed and well-defined ontology language, but also adequate support from reasoning tools. Ontology reasoning is a methodology for extracting and inferring knowledge from ontologies. Description Logic (DL)-based reasoners including *RacerPro*, *FaCT++*, and *Pellet* can efficiently perform reasoning over expressive OWL ontologies. However, these reasoners perform in-memory reasoning and are not particularly suitable for reasoning over ontologies with millions of instances such as those often needed for real-world applications such as healthcare systems.

Several approaches have been applied to improve the scalability of the reasoners. One of the most widely used approaches is database integration, i.e., utilizing secondary memory to increase efficiency. A number of reasoners such as OntMinD [5] and QuOnto [4] use database integration by directly mapping ontologies to databases. In this approach, ontologies are expressed in terms of UML class diagrams or/and ER diagrams and query rewriting techniques are used to perform reasoning over information stored in relational databases [10]. However, this approach restricts the expressivity of ontologies and supports only a small fragment of DL logic called DL-Lite [9]. DL-Lite is the maximal tractable fragment that supports efficient query answering using a relational database. So scalable reasoning with more expressive DL fragments is still a challenging problem. Another approach to improve the scalability of reasoners for more expressive ontologies is the logic programming-based approach. In this approach, an ontology is translated to a logic program, then inference algorithms for logic programs are used for reasoning. The main advantage of this approach is to reuse existing efficient inference algorithms and implementations, which are suitable for large ontologies. Logic programming-based approaches improve the scalability of the reasoning systems by handling large amounts of instances but still restrict the expressivity of ontologies [16].

In this paper, we present a scalable reasoning system, OwlOntDB, for OWL 2 RL ontologies. Here, by scalability, we refer the ability to perform reasoning over ontologies with large numbers of instances. The new standardization, OWL 2, has three profiles: OWL 2 EL - based on the EL^{++} Description Logic, OWL 2 QL - based on the DL-Lite family of Description Logics, and OWL 2 RL - inspired by pD^* and Description Logic Programs (DLP) [12]. Each profile exhibits a polynomial time complexity for ontological reasoning tasks. We choose OWL 2 RL because it offers a great deal of expressivity while being suitable for rule-based implementations. Grosof et al. [12] give a DLP mapping to translate OWL 1 ontologies to datalog programs to take advantage of logic programming-based algorithms to infer knowledge. In our hybrid approach, we extend the DLP mapping to accommodate the new features of OWL 2 RL, combine this with a mapping to a relational database to develop a restrictions checker to handle some OWL 2 RL axioms and concepts that cannot be handled by the logic programming-based approach, and then materialize all asserted and inferred knowledge from an ontology to a relational database. Our approach is a combination of the database mapping and the logic programming-based inferencing. However, instead of using the direct-mapping based approach to map OWL 2 RL ontologies to relational databases as in [10], we used a novel database-driven forward chaining approach to infer and store OWL 2 RL ontologies to relational databases.

The remainder of the paper is organized as follows. In section 2 we describe our scalable reasoning system, OwlOntDB. In section 3 we evaluate the performance of our system using two benchmark ontologies and a real-world ontology for healthcare. We discuss related work in section 4 and conclude in section 5.

2 A Scalable Reasoning System for Large ABoxes: OwlOntDB

We recall that OWL 2 is based on the family of Description Logics (DL) [6], a family of decidable fragments of first order logic. A DL-based ontology has two components: a TBox and an ABox. The TBox introduces vocabulary relevant to a domain and their semantics, while the ABox contains assertions about individuals using this vocabulary. Our reasoning system supports OWL 2 RL, which describes the domain of an ontology in terms of classes, properties, individuals, and datatypes and values. Individual names refer to elements of the domain; classes describe sets of individuals having similar characteristics; properties describe binary relationships between pairs of individuals. A property can be either an object property which links an individual to an individual, or a datatype property which links an individual to a data value. In OWL 2 RL, object properties can be functional, inverse functional, irreflexive, symmetric, asymmetric, or transitive; however, data properties can only be functional [20]. Note that the new features of OWL 2 RL not found in OWL 1 are qualified cardinality restrictions, irreflexive, and antisymmetric properties, and property chain inclusion axioms. The syntax of OWL 2 RL is asymmetric, i.e., the syntactic restrictions allowed for subclass expressions differ from those allowed for superclass expressions. For instance, an existential quantification to a class expression (ObjectSomeValuesFrom) is allowed only in subclass expressions whereas universal quantification to a class expression (ObjectAllValuesFrom) is allowed only in superclass expressions. These restrictions facilitate the rule-based implementation of reasoning systems for OWL 2 RL ontologies. Note that at present we assume the Unique Name Assumption (UNA) to translate OWL 2 RL ontologies into datalog programs. However, OWL 2 RL does not use the UNA i.e., it does not treat two different OWL 2 RL elements with different names as different. We are currently in the process of removing this limitation.

Ontological reasoning tasks are related either to the TBox, or to the ABox or to both the TBox and the ABox of an ontology. Here we focus on developing a scalable reasoner for reasoning tasks related to the ABox, namely ABox queries and mixed TBox and ABox queries. We use an existing DL-based reasoner to perform the TBox reasoning necessary to infer the complete subsumption

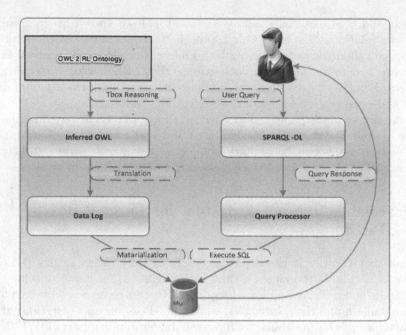

Fig. 1. The system architecture of OwlOntDB

relationship among classes (i.e., generate the class hierarchy). The overview of our system is found in Fig 1. OwlOntDB takes an OWL 2 RL ontology and materializes the datalog version of the classified ontology to the relational database using our technique which we refer to as a database-driven forward chaining and uses a modified SPARQL-DL as a query interface to extract knowledge from the database. The details of each step are explained in the following subsections.

2.1 Translation

Our approach to reasoning is to express inference tasks for the OWL 2 RL ontology in terms of inference tasks for the rule language datalog. Datalog is a simple rule language stemming from Prolog. In this step, we translate the classified ontology to a datalog programs using our extended DLP mapping. We use the OWL API to parse the classified OWL 2 RL ontology and extract all the logical axioms from the ontology. Then, we translate each logical axiom into its equivalent datalog rule(s). In OWL 2 RL, facts are described using ClassAssertions and ObjectPropertyAssertions/DataPropertyAssertions which correspond to DL axioms of the form $a : C$ and $\langle a, b \rangle : P$, respectively, where a and b are individuals, C is a class, and P is an object/data property. These assertions axioms are already in the datalog rule format with empty bodies. Translations of the OWL 2 RL axioms into datalog rules are given in Table 1. Their (straightforward) semantics may be found in [11].

Recall that we translate an ontology to a logic program in order to use the logic programming-based inference algorithm for ontology reasoning. However,

Table 1. Translation of OWL 2 RL axioms into datalog rules

OWL 2 RL Constructors	DL Syntax	Datalog Rule
ClassAssertions	$a : C$	$C(a)$
PropertyAssertion	$\langle a, b \rangle : P$	$P(a, b)$
SubClassOf	$C \sqsubseteq D$	$C(x) \to D(x)$
ObjectPropertyChain	$P \circ Q \sqsubseteq R$	$P(x, y) \wedge Q(y, z) \to R(x, z)$
EquivalentClasses	$C \equiv D$	$C(x) \to D(x), D(x) \to C(x)$
EquivalentProperties	$P \equiv Q$	$Q(x, y) \to P(x, y)$
		$P(x, y) \to Q(x, y)$
ObjectInverseOf	$P \equiv Q^{-}$	$P(x, y) \to Q(y, x)$
		$Q(y, x) \to P(x, y)$
TransitiveObjectProperty	$P^{+} \sqsubseteq P$	$P(x, y) \wedge P(y, z) \to P(x, z)$
SymmetricObjectProperty	$P \equiv P^{-}$	$P(x, y) \to P(y, x)$
Object/DataUnionOf	$C_1 \sqcup C_2 \sqsubseteq D$	$C_1(x) \to D(x), C_2(x) \to D(x)$
Object/DataIntersectionOf	$C \sqsubseteq D_1 \sqcap D_2$	$C(x) \to D_1(x), C(x) \to D_2(x)$
Object/DataSomeValuesFrom	$\exists P.C \sqsubseteq D$	$P(x, y) \wedge C(y) \to D(x)$
Object/DataAllValuesFrom	$C \sqsubseteq \forall P.D$	$C(x) \wedge P(x, y) \to D(y)$
Object/DataPropertyDomain	$\top \sqsubseteq \forall P^{-}.C$	$P(y, x) \to C(y)$
Object/DataPropertyRange	$\top \sqsubseteq \forall P.C$	$P(x, y) \to C(y)$

we can not handle OWL 2 RL concepts dealing with cardinality restrictions
- namely, maximum cardinality and minimum cardinality, and axioms dealing
with property restrictions - namely, functional, inverse functional, irreflexive,
asymmetric - using a logic programming-based approach. These concepts and
axioms impose certain restrictions over the object and data properties of an ontology and any violation of these restrictions results in an inconsistent ABox.
We developed a two-phase approach to the translation, using first an automated
translator to translate the ontology to datalog and then a restrictions checker to
check for ABox consistency with respect to the restriction concepts and axioms.
We represent each restriction concept/axiom by a datalog rule and then store
the restrictions of a property to a relational database by translating the datalog rule to an SQL statement. For each assertion the restrictions checker checks
whether it violates any restrictions. The datalog representations of the restriction concepts and axioms are given in Table 2. We illustrate this with a brief
example: Suppose we have a TBox axiom *IrreflexiveObjectProperty(hasSibling)*
(*hasSibling* is an irreflexive object property) and then we infer an ABox axiom
hasSibling(Bob, Bob). Now the ABox of the ontology will be inconsistent with
respect to the TBox axiom because *Bob* cannot be the sibling of himself (*irreflexivity*). We identify all violations according to the semantics of the axioms
listed in Table 2, where $n = 0$ or 1.

2.2 Materialization

Materialization [8] is an approach for inferring and storing implicit knowledge
from ontologies. If the ABox of an ontology is large and the query rate is high, the

Table 2. Datalog representation of the restrictions checker's concepts and axioms

MinimumCardinality	MaximumCardinality
$\geqslant nP.C$	$\leqslant nP.C$
$ObjectMinCardinality(n\ P\ C)$	$ObjectMaxCardinality(n\ P\ C)$
FunctionalProperty	InverseFunctionalProperty
$\top \sqsubseteq\ \leqslant 1\ P$	$\top \sqsubseteq\ \leqslant 1\ P^{-}$
$FunctionalObjectProperty(P)$	$InverseFunctionalObjectProperty(P)$
Irreflexive	Asymmetric
$\exists\ P.self \sqsubseteq \bot$	$P \sqsubseteq \neg P^{-}$
$IrreflexiveObjectProperty(P)$	$AsymmetricObjectProperty(P)$

materialization technique is faster than the approaches that perform reasoning during query evaluation. Materialization techniques are used in many scalable reasoners, including [5], [21] and [18]. In our materialization approach, we use the forward-chaining method to infer implicit knowledge and a relational database to store information. In this section, we give a formal representation of the datalog version of the translated ontology by an abstract syntax, explain how a datalog rule can be translated to an SQL statement, and discuss the inferencing over datalog programs.

The abstract syntax for our datalog program is given in Listing 1.1 using a BNF. In this notation, the terminals are quoted, the non-terminals are not quoted, alternatives are separated by vertical bars, and components that can occur zero or more times are enclosed by braces followed by a superscript asterisk symbol ({...}*). A class atom represented by *class(i-object)* in the BNF consists of a class and a single argument representing an individual. For example, an atom *Person(x)* holds if x is an instance of the class *Person*. Similarly, an individual property atom represented by *ObjectProperty(i-object,i-object)* consists of an object property and two arguments representing individuals. For example, an atom *hasDog(x,y)* holds if x is related to y by property *hasDog*. A functional object property such as *hasMother* is encoded as *FunctionalObjectProperty (hasMother)*. If an atom is a ground fact, i.e., there are no variables in its argument list, we call it a restrictive atom, because such an atom is restricted to appear only in the head of a datalog rule.

As we already mentioned, storing asserted and inferred information is part of materialization and to achieve this, we translate each datalog rule to an equivalent SQL statement. We use a database structure adapted from [18] which has 33 relational tables to store OWL 2 RL ontologies. The structure uses a metamapping approach, putting all the Class assertions into one table, all the Object Property assertions into a second table and all the Data Property assertions into a third table, rather than using a separate table for each predicate. Extensions of the database corresponding to extensions of an ontology are then easy to make. A fragment of the database structure is given in Figure 2 where some tables including their column names are shown. An arrow between two tables represents a referential constraint (functional dependency) between the tables. Referential constraints are also known as foreign keys.

```
Program ::=Rule {Rule}*
Rule ::= Head | Head '←' Body
Head ::= Atom | RestrictedAtom
Body ::= Atom{∧ Atom}*
Atom ::= Class '(' i-object ')'
       | ObjectProperty '(' i-object ',' i-object ')'
       | DataProperty '(' i-object ',' d-object ')'

RestrictedAtom ::= 'InverseObjectProperty(' PropertyID ',' PropertyID')'
                 | 'FunctionalObjectProperty(' PropertyID ')'
                 | 'InverseFunctionalObjectProperty(' PropertyID ')'
                 | 'SymmetricObjectProperty(' PropertyID ')'
                 | 'AsymmetricObjectProperty(' PropertyID ')'
                 | 'TransitiveObjectProperty(' PropertyID ')'
                 | 'IrreflexiveObjectProperty(' PropertyID ')'
                 | 'FunctionalDataProperty(' PropertyID ')'
                 | 'ObjectMinCardinality(' n PropertyID ClassID ')'
                 | 'ObjectMaxCardinality(' n PropertyID ClassID')'
                 | 'ObjectPropertyDomain(' ClassID ')'
                 | 'ObjectPropertyRange(' ClassID ')'
                 | 'DataPropertyDomain(' ClassID ')'
                 | 'DataPropertyRange(' ClassID ')'

i-object ::= i-variable | individualID
d-object ::= d-variable | dataLiteral
i-variable ::= 'I-variable(' URIreference ')'
d-variable ::= 'D-variable(' URIreference ')'
```

Listing 1.1. Abstract syntax for datalog programs

In our datalog program, a datalog rule has one of the following forms

$$head(h_1, \ldots h_n) \tag{1}$$

$$head(h_1, \ldots h_n) \leftarrow body(b_1, \ldots, b_n) \tag{2}$$

$$head(h_1, \ldots h_n) \leftarrow body_0(b_1, \ldots, b_n) \wedge \ldots \wedge body_n(b_1, \ldots, b_n) \tag{3}$$

Datalog rules are closely related to operations in relational algebra, and the foundation of SQL is also relational algebra. Analogies between datalog and relational query languages such as SQL are well known and well studied [3]. We translate the three kinds of datalog rules to their corresponding SQL statements as follows:

```
(1) INSERT INTO <Table1> VALUES ( h₁,...hₙ)
(2) INSERT INTO <Table1> SELECT
                <Projectors> FROM <Tables> WHERE <SELECTORS>
(3) INSERT INTO <Table1> SELECT <Projectors>
         FROM <Table2> JOIN ... JOIN <TableN> WHERE <SELECTORS>
```

We use an exhaustive forward-chaining approach to infer implicit knowledge, i.e., for each class/property assertion a forward-chaining is performed. This is a novel database-driven forward chaining. We first translate all the ABox facts and the TBox rules to their corresponding SQL statements. Executing the SQL statements corresponding to the ABox stores these facts into a relational database. For each fact we determine the rules relevant for forward chaining. Executing

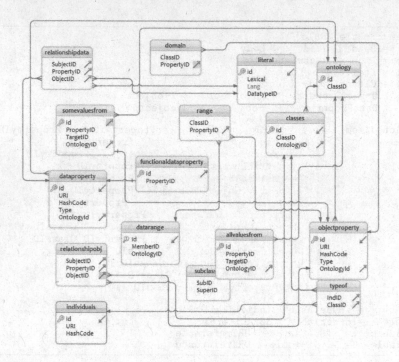

Fig. 2. A fragment of the database schema

the SQL statements for these rules stores new (inferred) facts into the database. Before storing any inferred information, we check whether it violates any restrictions listed in Table 2 by executing SQL statements corresponding to the restrictions checker's axioms and concepts.

Note that the W3C also recommends a set of rules corresponding to the OWL 2 RL profile. However, we are using set of datalog rules because the complexity of forward-chaining approach over datalog programs is polynomial and the relationship between datalog and SQL facilitates our database-driven forward-chaining approach.

Our algorithm, $Materialize(\mathcal{R}, \mathcal{F})$, takes the datalog version of the OWL 2 RL ontology, and performs forward chaining to infer implicit knowledge. The algorithm $Materialize(\mathcal{R}, \mathcal{F})$ (Line 1 - 8) invokes the procedure $Consequences(r, \mathcal{F})$ to populate the relational database by asserted ABox facts and to select a set of firable rules to perform database-driven forward-chaining. The $Consequences(r, \mathcal{F})$ (Line 1 -4) first checks whether the first argument is a rule or a fact. If it is a fact, then it converts to it an equivalent SQL statement and executes the SQL statement to store the asserted or inferred facts into the database. If the argument is not a fact (Line 5 - 9), this procedure checks whether the rule is firable. A firable rule is enabled if the body predicates of the rule are matched by asserted or inferred facts. (Note we do not add inferred facts to F, as our algorithm is not main-memory-based. Rather the $isFirable(r)$ function accesses (asserted and inferred) facts from the database.) After getting the set of firable rules, the

Materialize($\mathcal{R}$, $\mathcal{F}$) algorithm, (Line 7), translates each rule to its equivalent SQL statement and translates all others datalog rules (i.e., not firable rules) to their equivalent SQL statements in (Line 10 -11). Before storing inferred facts by executing all the SQL statements, the *checkRestriction*(s) (Line 12) method checks whether any assertion violates any restrictions and if not, it allows the execution of the associated SQL statement by *executeSQL*(s) to store the information in a relational database, otherwise it raises an exception message about the inconsistency of the ABox (Line 11 - 13). For example, if *hasMother*(x, y) is a functional object property, the restrictions checker queries the relational database to check whether x is connected to more than one different y. Full details of the *checkRestriction*(s) method may be found in [11].

Algorithm 1. Materialize($\mathcal{R}$, $\mathcal{F}$) - materialize a datalog program into the database

---

Data: $\mathcal{R}$- set of datalog rules $\mathcal{F}$- set of ABox facts
Result: $\mathcal{S}$- set of SQL statements.

1 **repeat**
2   *inferred* $\Leftarrow$ *false*
3   **for** $\forall\ r\ \in\ \mathcal{R}$ **do**
4   **for** $\forall\ f\ \in\ Consequences(r,\ \mathcal{F})$ **do**
5   **if** $f \notin \mathcal{F}$ **then**
6   *inferred* $\Leftarrow$ *true*
7              $\mathcal{S} \Leftarrow$ *datalogToSQL*(f)

8 **until** ! *inferred*
9 **for** $\forall\ r\ \in\ \mathcal{R}$ **do**
10     $\mathcal{S} \Leftarrow$ *datalogToSQL*(r)

11 **for** $\forall\ s\ \in\ S$ **do**
12   **if** *checkRestriction*(s) **then**
13   *executeSQL*(s)

2.3 Query Processing

In this subsection, we describe a query interface to extract materialized knowledge from the database. SPARQL [25] is a W3C recommendation for querying RDF graphs. An RDF graph is a collection of *(subject, predicate, object)* triples. We cannot use SPARQL as it exists as a query language for OWL 2 RL for two reasons. First, it is based on the triple patterns of RDF graphs, but RDF triple patterns do not match the well-defined OWL 2 RL syntax, so a modified version of SPARQL is necessary. Second, in our framework, we materialize ontologies to relational databases. So we need a modified version of SPARQL to retrieve data from relational databases.

SQL, the query language for relational databases, includes support for large data-storage, efficient indexing schemes, and query optimization. If we directly

---

Procedure Consequences$(r, \mathcal{F})$ - recursively applied for all the predicates of a rule body to derive the consequence

---

Data: r - a datalog rule, $\mathcal{F}$- set of ABox facts.

1 **if** r *is a fact* **then**
2     $datalogToSQL(r)$
3     $executeSQL(s)$
4   **return** r

5 $inferred \Leftarrow \emptyset$
6 **for** $\forall f \in \mathcal{F}$ **do**
7   **if** $isFirable(r)$ **then**
8        $inferred \Leftarrow inferred \cup r$

9 **return** $inferred$

---

use SQL to extract knowledge from materialized ontologies, then users have to learn the underlying relational schemas. Many real-world semantic web-based applications need to extract data from both relational sources and ontologies. So a uniform query language is necessary for accessing both structured data (e.g., from relational databases) and semi-structured data (e.g., RDF triples, OWL ontologies).

In order to use SPARQL for querying ontologies based on OWL 1, Sirin and Parsia [27] designed a query language by modifying SPARQL called SPARQL-DL, a substantial subset of SPARQL, by mapping RDF triple patterns using OWL 1 DL semantics. Therefore, SPARQL-DL supports only the semantics of OWL 1 ontologies. The SPARQL-DL API [2] supports a query language, which we will refer to as SPARQL-DL$_E$, for OWL 2 ontologies (including OWL 2 RL ontologies). However, the SPARQL-DL API is built to interface with main-memory-based OWL 2 reasoners, so we need some modifications to support queries over the relational database-based reasoner. In this subsection, we describe the semantics of SPARQL-DL$_E$ and explain our modifications.

The Semantics of SPARQL-DL$_E$. SPARQL-DL$_E$ is an expressive query language that can combine TBox and ABox queries. Here we briefly describe the semantics of SPARQL-DL$_E$ which we extended from [27].

Let $\mathcal{O}$ be an OWL 2 ontology, let $V_O = (\mathcal{V}_{cls}, \mathcal{V}_{op}, \mathcal{V}_{dp}, \mathcal{V}_{ind}, \mathcal{V}_D, \mathcal{V}_{lit})$ be a vocabulary for $\mathcal{O}$ and let $I = (\Delta^I, {}^{\cdot I})$ be an interpretation for $\mathcal{O}$. The list of SPARQL-DL query atoms for OWL 1 and their corresponding semantics may be found in [27]. Two new query atoms are required to deal with OWL 2: Reflexive(p) and Irreflexive(p). Their semantics is given in Table 3. Here $a_{(i)} \in \mathcal{V}_{uri} \cup \mathcal{V}_{var} \cup \mathcal{V}_{bnode}$, $d \in \mathcal{V}_{uri} \cup \mathcal{V}_{var} \cup \mathcal{V}_{bnode} \cup \mathcal{V}_{lit}$, $C_{(i)} \in \mathcal{V}_{var} \cup \mathcal{S}_c$, $p_{(i)} \in \mathcal{V}_{uri} \cup \mathcal{V}_{var}$, $\mathcal{V}_{cls}$ is the set of classes, $\mathcal{V}_{op}$ is the set of object properties, $\mathcal{V}_{dp}$ is the set of data properties, $\mathcal{V}_{ind}$ is the set of individuals, $\mathcal{V}_{lit}$ is the set of literals and $\mathcal{V}_D$ is the set of data types of $\mathcal{O}$. Note that OWL 2 RL does not include reflexivity, so our reasoning system does not support queries involving reflexive properties.

Table 3. Satisfaction of a SPARQL-DL$_E$ query atom with respect to an interpretation

Query atom q	$\mathcal{I} \models_\delta q$ if
$Type(a, C)$	$\delta(a) \in C^\mathcal{I}$
$Reflexive(p)$	$< a, b > \in p^\mathcal{I}$ implies $a = b$
$Irreflexive(p)$	$< a, b > \in p^\mathcal{I}$ implies $a \neq b$

An evaluation $\delta : \mathcal{V}_{ind} \cup \mathcal{V}_{bnode} \cup \mathcal{V}_{lit} \rightarrow \Delta^\mathcal{I}$ is a mapping from the individual names, blank nodes, and literals used in the query to the elements of the interpretation domain $\Delta^\mathcal{I}$ subject to the requirement $\delta(a) = a^\mathcal{I}$ if $a \in \mathcal{V}_{ind}$ or $a \in \mathcal{V}_{lit}$. The interpretation $\mathcal{I}$ satisfies a query atom q, $\mathcal{I} \models_\delta q$, if q is compatible with the corresponding condition for the query atom. $\mathcal{I}$ satisfies a query $Q = q_1 \wedge \ldots \wedge q_n$. w.r.t. an evaluation δ **iff** $\mathcal{I} \models_\delta q_i$ for every $i = 1, \ldots, n$.

A solution to a query Q is a mapping $\mu : \mathcal{V}_{var} \rightarrow \mathcal{V}_{cls} \cup \mathcal{V}_{op} \cup \mathcal{V}_{dp} \cup \mathcal{V}_{lit}$ such that when all the variables in Q are substituted with the corresponding value from μ we get a ground query $\mu(Q)$ (i.e., an atom having no variables) compatible with $\mathcal{V}_\mathcal{O}$ and $\mathcal{O} \models \mu(Q)$.

Implementation of SPARQL-DL$_E$ in OwlOntDB. We modified the SPARQL-DL API to extract knowledge from the relational database and implemented it in our system. The SPARQL-DL API is built on top of the OWL API [15]. The SPARQL-DL API was designed in such a way that it can answer mixed TBox and ABox queries by invoking interfaces, such as $allC(\mathcal{O})$, $allDP(\mathcal{O})$, $allOP(\mathcal{O})$, $allI(\mathcal{O})$, etc., provided by the ontology reasoner. We modified these interfaces (see the full list of interfaces that required modification below) so that this API can evaluate queries using our persistent reasoning system.

1. $allC(\mathcal{O})$, $allDP(\mathcal{O})$, $allOP(\mathcal{O})$, $allI(\mathcal{O})$ return all classes, data properties, object properties, and individuals, respectively, defined in $\mathcal{O}$.
2. $subC(\mathcal{O}, \mathcal{C})$, $supC(\mathcal{O}, \mathcal{C})$, $eqC(\mathcal{O}, \mathcal{C})$ return all sub classes, super classes, and equivalent classes, respectively, of class C in $\mathcal{O}$.
3. $subOP(\mathcal{O}, \mathcal{P})$, $supOP(\mathcal{O}, \mathcal{P})$, $eqOP(\mathcal{O}, \mathcal{P})$, $subDP(\mathcal{O}, \mathcal{P})$, $supDP(\mathcal{O}, \mathcal{P})$, $eq DP(\mathcal{O}, \mathcal{P})$ return all sub object properties, super object properties, equivalent object properties, sub data properties, super data properties, and equivalent data properties, respectively, of properties p in $\mathcal{O}$.
4. $en(\mathcal{O}, q)$ checks whether $\mathcal{O} \models q$ for a SPARQL-DL$_E$ atom q.

Recall we stored asserted and inferred information from ontologies into databases. Therefore, we need an SQL query for each interface described in (1)-(3) to retrieve relevant information from corresponding tables of the relational database. For example, the SQL queries for $subC(\mathcal{O}, \mathcal{C})$ and $supOP(\mathcal{O}, \mathcal{P})$ are:

```
SELECT SubID FROM SubClassOf WHERE SuperID = C
SELECT SuperPropertyID FROM SuperPropertyOf WHERE SubPropertyID = P
```

The SQL queries retrieve all subclasses for a given class and all super properties for a given object property, respectively. The query given in 4. is evaluated by the

SPARQL-DL API by invoking the appropriate interfaces discussed in 1.-3. For instance, if we consider the query $q = SubClassOf('' Person'', c)$, the SPARQL-DL API will invoke the interface $subC(\mathcal{O}, Person)$ to retrieve all the subclasses of "Person" from the database.

3   Evaluation

We evaluated OwlOntDB using an OWL 2 RL pain management ontology constructed from the guidelines for the management of cancer related pain in adults, which provides a standard approach in assessing and managing cancer related pain in adults across Nova Scotia, Canada [7]. We evaluated OwlOntDB using this pain ontology because there are no widely accepted benchmarks for OWL 2. In [22], the authors discussed this problem and identified that while there are some ontologies that can be used as standards for testing TBox reasoning, there are no such standards for ABox reasoning. Evaluation was done on a laptop computer with 2.4 GHz Intel Core 2 Duo processor, 4 GB of RAM running Mac OS X version 10.6.8.

We use the pain management ontology [26] that includes the terminology and concepts of health and medicine used in the Guysborough Antigonish Strait Health Authority (GASHA) and some terms from SNOMED-CT [1], ICNP [14], and the guidelines for cancer pain treatment. A fragment of the pain management ontology is depicted in Figure 3. Our ontology includes several classes including *Pain*, *Person*, *Patient*, *PainIntensityType*, *SpecialPainProblem*, *SideEffects*; some object properties including *hasPainIntensity*, *Domain:Pain*, *Range:PainInt- ensity-Type*, and data properties including *hasPainLevel*, *Domain :Pain*, *Range:xs- d:int*, inverse object properties such as *isFeeling* and *isFeltBy*, and functional object properties including *hasPainLevel*, i.e., each pain level belongs to an instance of *Pain* class. We also use propositional connectives to create complex class expressions (e.g., persons who feel pain are patients, in DL $Person \sqcap \exists isFeeling.Pain \sqsubseteq Patient$). We developed a data generator similar to that developed for the LUBM benchmark [13] to synthetically generate large numbers of instances for the pain management ontology. We generated five test datasets, PM_{250}, PM_{500}, PM_{1000}, PM_{2000}, and PM_{3000}, where the number of patients n = 250, 500, 1000, 2000, and 3000, respectively, and evaluated the following two queries to evaluate the performance of our system. The SPARQL-DL$_E$ formulation of each query appears below its natural language formulation.

PM Q_1. *Determine the medication information of all patients who feel "Mucositis" pain.*

```
PREFIX pm: <http://logic.stfx.ca/ontologies/PainOntology.owl#>
  SELECT ?i ?j WHERE {
  Type(?i,pm:Patient), PropertyValue(?i, pm:isFeeling, pm:MucositisPain),
    PropertyValue(?i, pm:hasMedication, ?j) }
```

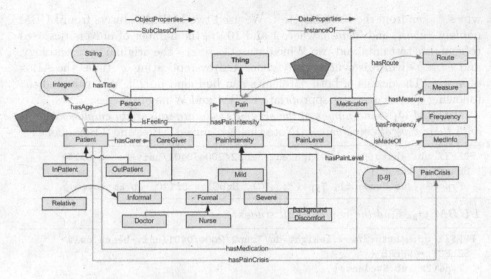

Fig. 3. A fragment of the pain management ontology

PM Q_2. *Find the names of those relatives (of patients) who serve as informal care givers.*

```
PREFIX pm: <http://logic.stfx.ca/ontologies/PainOntology.owl#>
    SELECT ?i ?j WHERE {
    Type(?i,pm:Patient), PropertyValue(?i, pm:hasCarer , ?j),
        SubClassOf(?j, pm:Relative) }
```

The first query is a conjunctive ABox query and the second query is a conjunctive mixed TBox and ABox query. We evaluated these queries over the corresponding ontologies using OwlOntDB and also using two highly optimized in-memory reasoners *Pellet* and *RacerPro* 2.0. Our goal is to show that in-memory reasoners cannot deal with ontologies with large ABoxes. The OwlOntDB materializes the information to a database, so it needs an initial processing before query evaluation. The initial processing time (i.e., materialization time) for five datasets required for OwlOntDB and total number of axioms in each ontology are given in Table 4.

Table 4. Time required for materialization for the PM ontology

	PM_{250}	PM_{500}	PM_{1000}	PM_{2000}	PM_{3000}
No. of Axioms	20344	40396	77600	156308	231555
Time (sec.)	20.71	45.94	90.34	263.24	345.28

We also evaluated our system using two well-known benchmark ontologies for OWL 1: LUBM - an ontology about organizational structures of universities developed to test the performance of ontology management and reasoning systems [1], and the Wine ontology - an ontology containing a classification of

---

[1] http://swat.cse.lehigh.edu/downloads/index.html

wines, taken from the KAON2 site [2]. We used two LUBM datasets from LUBM namely, $lubm_1$, and $lubm_{10}$, where 1 and 10 are the number of universities used to generate test data and two Wine datasets $wine_1$ - the original wine ontology, and $wine_5$ - which is synthetically generated by replicating 2^5 times the ABox of $wine_1$. The details of both ontologies can be found in [22]. We evaluated the following queries over the appropriate LUBM and Wine ontologies:

LUBM Q_1. *Find names of the students who are university employees along with their type of employment.* (Note this is a mixed ABox and TBox query.)

```
PREFIX ub: <http://www.lehigh.edu/~zhp2/2004/0401/univ-bench.owl#>
SELECT * WHERE {
  Type(?x, ub:Student), Type(?x, ?C), SubClassOf(?C, ub:Employee)}
```

LUBM Q_2. *Find the names of all students.*

```
PREFIX ub: <http://www.lehigh.edu/~zhp2/2004/0401/univ-bench.owl#>
SELECT * WHERE {
  Type(?x, ub:Student)}
```

Wine Q_1 *Determine all instances of "AmericanWine".*

```
PREFIX wine: <http://www.w3.org/TR/2003/PR-owl-guide-20031209/wine#>
SELECT ?i WHERE {
  Type(?i, wine:AmericanWine)}
```

Wine Q_2 *Determine all the instances of wine which are "Dry".*

```
PREFIX wine: <http://www.w3.org/TR/2003/PR-owl-guide-20031209/wine#>
SELECT ?i WHERE {
  Type(?i,?x), SubClassOf(?x, wine:DryWine) }
```

The materialization time for the LUBM and Wine ontologies required for OwlOntDB and total number of axioms in each ontology are given in Table 5.

Table 5. Time required for materialization for the LUBM and Wine ontologies

	$LUBM_1$	$LUBM_{10}$	$Wine_1$	$Wine_5$
No. of Axioms	84562	1316410	649	5576
Time (sec.)	117.58	830.53	21.422	217.5

The query evaluation time for *Pellet*, *RacerPro*, and OwlOntDB is given in Table 6. Standard tableau-based reasoners support more expressive fragments of DL and efficiently perform reasoning over ontologies with small ABoxes. From our experiments, we found that for ontologies with large ABoxes, our reasoning outperformed its tableau counterpart. Although we first used a tableau-based DL reasoner for the TBox reasoning required for classification, we get better performance for the query evaluation than these tableau-based reasoners because we first materialized the inferred information into a database. After the

---

[2] http://kaon2.semanticweb.org/download/test_ontologies.zip

Table 6. A comparison of query answering times (in seconds). "-" means that the reasoner failed to return the result and "..." means that the reasoner does not support the query. Note that *RacerPro* supports only TBox queries, a limitation not due to in-memory problems but due to the nature of *RacerPro*.

	Q_1			Q_2		
	Pellet	RacerPro	OwlOntDB	Pellet	RacerPro	OwlOntDB
PM_{250}	41.65	27	7.53	65.85	...	9.79
PM_{500}	91.83	70	11.71	127.038	...	14.89
PM_{1000}	179.50	105.5	16.89	259.678	...	19.01
PM_{2000}	718.18	225	20.78	959.32	...	23.21
PM_{3000}	-	430	29.21	-	...	34.01
$LUBM_1$	129.02	...	3.43	127	73	0.79
$LUBM_{10}$	-	...	29.07	-	-	15.03
$Wine_1$	2.95	24	0.047	2.9	...	0.11
$Wine_5$	6.08	37	0.3435	386.59	...	1.171

materialization, reasoning over a materialized ontology is simply an SQL query into a relational database. Main-memory based reasoners perform inferencing for each query, so they take a longer time when the ABox is large. Indeed, we can see from the Table 6 that we do not get any query result from either *Pellet* or *RacerPro* for a large ontology like $LUBM_{10}$, but, the query response time for this ontology using our OwlOntDB is very low. The disadvantage of the materialization technique is that it takes a long time initially to materialize the ontology.

Recall we use a standard DL reasoner for the TBox reasoning which creates a complete class hierarchy if the corresponding TBox is consistent. Therefore, OwlOntDB is complete for TBox reasoning. The ABox reasoning is based on a database-driven forward chaining approach. The empirical completeness of ABox reasoning was checked by comparing the ABox reasoning results with the results of the OWL 2 reasoners *Pellet* and *RacerPro*. A similar empirical approach is used in [23], to compare their in-memory-based OWL 2 RL reasoners with Hermit. While efficient for the TBox reasoning, their in-memory-based implementation performed poorly on ontologies with large ABoxes. We are still working on the algorithm to deal with the situation where the set of axioms is cyclic; currently our algorithm may not terminate if the set of axioms is cyclic.

4   Related Work

There has recently been considerable interest in developing scalable persistent reasoning systems for Semantic Web applications. The integration of relational databases and DL-based reasoners has been realized in many research initiatives including [18], [29], [4]. Most scalable reasoning systems such as Minerva [29], SOAR [18], and DLDB2 [24] combine existing DL reasoners with logic programming-based approaches. However, these reasoners are based on DLP, providing only incomplete coverage of OWL 2 RL reasoning. We use a 2-phase approach to deal with all OWL 2 RL axioms.

OWLIM [16] is an in-memory reasoner. It also uses the logic programming based approach (i.e., forward-chaining for inferencing) and focuses only on the DLP fragment, hence it covers a subset of OWL 2 RL. Another logic programming-based DL reasoner is KAON2 [21]. In KAON2, the ontology is translated into a logic program and then it is materialized into a deductive database for querying and storing the information. This approach is similar to our approach, except we develop a scalable reasoner for OWL 2 RL, a more expressive fragment than that supported by KAON2, and materialize the information to a relational database rather than to a deductive database.

Another database-driven reasoning system is Orel [17], which covers the full profile of OWL 2 RL as well as the OWL 2 EL profile, using an algorithm based on DLP. However, this system supports only TBox reasoning; it does not support (conjunctive) query answering (i.e., ABox reasoning). Another limitation of this system is that it does not support a standard query language for the extraction of knowledge from materialized ontologies, therefore, users have to know the detailed structure of the underlying database schema to extract knowledge using SQL. To extract knowledge from the database OwlOntDB supports SPARQL-DL_E, so users of our system have to know only about the ontology.

DLEJena [19] is an OWL 2 RL reasoner that also combines a forward-chaining-based rule engine Jena and a DL reasoner *Pellet*. It supports a practical subset of OWL 2 RL. A pair of OWL 2 RL reasoners is described in recent work, [23] using two existing rule systems Jess and Drools. However, these reasoners are all in-memory-based reasoners; they are not scalable: they cannot handle ontologies with large ABoxes. We could not find any scalable OWL 2 RL reasoners to use for comparison with our approach.

5   Conclusion and Future Work

Scalable reasoning is crucial for the development of large-scale ontology-driven applications. In this paper, we propose a practical scalable ontology reasoning approach. The combination of DL reasoners with logic-based inferencing using datalog exploits the particular advantages of each method in order to support expressive ontologies, such as those which use OWL 2 RL in their TBoxes, and large ABoxes. Logic-based approaches give us scalable reasoning strategies, and database systems are a well-known technology for handling large amounts of data. We develop a hybrid approach by applying database-driven forward chaining approach over logic-based translated ontologies that allows us to perform scalable reasoning over ontologies with large ABoxes. There is a number of advantages and disadvantage for materialization techniques. However, they are good for many applications where query answering is more frequent and updating is less frequent.

Our approach is still preliminary and some improvements can be made. One of the future directions to improve our system is to remove the Unique Name

Assumption (UNA) because UNA is not made in OWL 2 semantics. The initial processing time for the materialization is very high. Parallel and distributed computing may be applied to reduce the materialization time. However, this will not be fast enough for applications that require frequent update and real-time query answering, such as healthcare applications, where ontologies are used to drive decision support systems. The current strategy is to rematerialize the whole ontology if the ontology is updated, but this brings a heavy overhead as the time required for materialization must be added to the time for query-answering. Incremental materialization is anticipated to be an efficient solution for the update problem. We are working to reduce materialization time by replacing our exhaustive forward chaining inferencing approach by an incremental approach that rematerializes relevant axioms. We note that *Pellet* supports incremental materialization but only for concept assertions. There are also some works in deductive database areas for incremental maintenance of truth in materialization [28]; a further investigation can be made to check whether these techniques can be used for relational databases. Efficient handling of frequent updates in an ontology with large number of instances is an important aspect of developing large-scale ontology-driven systems such as healthcare systems.

Acknowledgments. This work is supported by an NSERC Discovery Grant, an NSERC Industrial Post Graduate Fellowship and ACOA. We would like to thank Fazle Rabbi for the help to develop benchmark data generator, Jocelyne Faddoul and Fazle Rabbi for support on *RacerPro* and Rachel Embree and Mary Heather Jewers for the fruitful discussions about ontologies and the guidelines for the management of cancer related pain in adults. We thank the anonymous referees for their comments and corrections.

References

1. SNOMED-CT Systematized Nomenclature of Medicine-Clinical Terms (2007), http://www.ihtsdo.org/snomed-ct/
2. SPARQL-DL API (2011), http://www.derivo.de/en/resources/sparql-dl-api/
3. Abiteboul, S., Hull, R., Vianu, V.: Foundations of Databases. Addison-Wesley (1995)
4. Acciarri, A., Calvanese, D., Giacomo, G.D., Lembo, D., Lenzerini, M., Palmieri, M., Rosati, R.: QuOnto: Querying Ontologies. In: Veloso, M.M., Kambhampati, S. (eds.) AAAI, pp. 1670–1671. AAAI Press/The MIT Press (2005)
5. Al-Jadir, L., Parent, C., Spaccapietra, S.: Reasoning with large ontologies stored in relational databases: The OntoMinD approach. Data & Knowledge Engineering 69(11), 1158–1180 (2010)
6. Baader, F., McGuinness, D.L., Nardi, D., Patel-Schneider, P.F. (eds.): The Description Logic Handbook: Theory, Implementation, and Applications. Cambridge University Press (2003)
7. Broadfield, L., Banerjee, S., Jewers, H., Pollett, A.J., Simpson, J.: Guidelines for the management of cancer-related pain in adults. Supportive care cancer site team, cancer care Nova Scotia, Canada (2005)
8. Broekstra, J.: Storage, Querying and Inferencing for Semantic Web Languages. Ph.D. thesis, VU Amsterdam (2005)

9. Calvanese, D., Giacomo, G., Lembo, D., Lenzerini, M., Rosati, R.: Tractable reasoning and efficient query answering in description logics: The DL-Lite Family. Journal of Automated Reasoning 39, 385–429 (2007)
10. Calvanese, D., De Giacomo, G., Lembo, D., Lenzerini, M., Poggi, A., Rodriguez-Muro, M., Rosati, R.: Ontologies and Databases: The *DL-Lite* Approach. In: Tessaris, S., Franconi, E., Eiter, T., Gutierrez, C., Handschuh, S., Rousset, M.-C., Schmidt, R.A. (eds.) Reasoning Web 2009. LNCS, vol. 5689, pp. 255–356. Springer, Heidelberg (2009)
11. Faruqui, R.U.: Scalable reasoning over large ontologies. MSc thesis, St. Francis Xavier University (2012), http://logic.stfx.ca/thesis/
12. Grosof, B.N., Horrocks, I., Volz, R., Decker, S.: Description logic programs: Combining logic programs with description logic. In: Proceedings of the 12th International Conference on World Wide Web, pp. 48–57. ACM Press (2003)
13. Guo, Y., Pan, Z., Heflin, J.: LUBM: A benchmark for OWL knowledge base systems. J. Web Sem. 3(2-3), 158–182 (2005)
14. Hardiker, N., Coenen, A.: A formal foundation for ICNP. Journal of Stud. Health Technol. Inform. 122, 705–709 (2006)
15. Horridge, M., Bechhofer, S.: The OWL API: A java API for working with OWL 2 Ontologies. In: 6th OWL Experienced and Directions Workshop (OWLED) (October 2009)
16. Kiryakov, A., Ognyanov, D., Manov, D.: OWLIM - A Pragmatic Semantic Repository for OWL. In: Dean, M., Guo, Y., Jun, W., Kaschek, R., Krishnaswamy, S., Pan, Z., Sheng, Q.Z. (eds.) WISE 2005 Workshops. LNCS, vol. 3807, pp. 182–192. Springer, Heidelberg (2005)
17. Krötzsch, M., Mehdi, A., Rudolph, S.: Orel: Database-Driven reasoning for OWL 2 Profiles. In: 23rd Int. Workshop on Description Logics (DL 2010), pp. 114–124 (2010)
18. Lu, J., Ma, L., Zhang, L., Brunner, J.S., Wang, C., Pan, Y., Yu, Y.: SOR: a practical system for ontology storage, reasoning and search. In: Proceedings of the 33rd International Conference on Very Large Data Bases, VLDB 2007, pp. 1402–1405. VLDB Endowment (2007)
19. Meditskos, G., Bassiliades, N.: DLEJena: A practical forward-chaining OWL 2 RL reasoner combining Jena and Pellet. Web Semant. 8(1), 89–94 (2010), http://dx.doi.org/10.1016/j.websem.2009.11.001
20. Motik, B., Grau, B., Horrocks, I., Wu, Z., Fokoue, A., Lutz, C.: OWL 2 Web Ontology Language: Profiles, W3C Recommendation (October 2009), http://www.w3.org/TR/owl2-profiles/
21. Motik, B.: KAON2 - Scalable Reasoning over Ontologies with Large Data Sets. ERCIM News 2008(72) (2008)
22. Motik, B., Sattler, U.: A Comparison of Reasoning Techniques for Querying Large Description Logic ABoxes. In: Hermann, M., Voronkov, A. (eds.) LPAR 2006. LNCS (LNAI), vol. 4246, pp. 227–241. Springer, Heidelberg (2006)
23. O'Connor, M.J., Das, A.: A Pair of OWL 2 RL Reasoners. In: Klinov, P., Horridge, M. (eds.) OWLED. CEUR Workshop Proceedings, vol. 849. CEUR-WS.org (2012)
24. Pan, Z., Zhang, X., Heflin, J.: DLDB2: A Scalable Multi-perspective Semantic Web Repository. In: Web Intelligence, pp. 489–495. IEEE (2008)
25. Prud'hommeaux, E., Seaborne, A.: SPARQL Query Language for RDF. W3C Recommendation (2008), http://www.w3.org/TR/rdf-sparql-query/
26. Rakib, A., Faruqui, R.U., MacCaull, W.: Verifying resource requirements for ontology-driven rule-based agents. In: Lukasiewicz, T., Sali, A. (eds.) FoIKS 2012. LNCS, vol. 7153, pp. 312–331. Springer, Heidelberg (2012)

27. Sirin, E., Parsia, B.: SPARQL-DL: Sparql query for OWL-DL. In: 3rd OWL Experiences and Directions Workshop (OWLED 2007) (2007)
28. Volz, R., Staab, S., Motik, B.: Incrementally Maintaining Materializations of Ontologies Stored in Logic Databases. In: Spaccapietra, S., Bertino, E., Jajodia, S., King, R., McLeod, D., Orlowska, M.E., Strous, L. (eds.) Journal on Data Semantics II. LNCS, vol. 3360, pp. 1–34. Springer, Heidelberg (2005)
29. Zhou, J., Ma, L., Liu, Q., Zhang, L., Yu, Y., Pan, Y.: Minerva: A Scalable OWL Ontology Storage and Inference System. In: Mizoguchi, R., Shi, Z.-Z., Giunchiglia, F. (eds.) ASWC 2006. LNCS, vol. 4185, pp. 429–443. Springer, Heidelberg (2006)

Trustworthy Pervasive Healthcare Services via Multiparty Session Types

Anders S. Henriksen[1], Lasse Nielsen[1], Thomas T. Hildebrandt[2], Nobuko Yoshida[3], and Fritz Henglein[1]

[1] University of Copenhagen
{starcke,lnielsen,henglein}@diku.dk
[2] IT University of Copenhagen
hilde@itu.dk
[3] Imperial College London
yoshida@doc.ic.ac.uk

Abstract. This paper proposes a new theory of *multiparty session types* extended with *propositional assertions* and *symmetric sum types* for modelling collaborative distributed workflows. Multiparty session types statically guarantee that workflows are type-safe and deadlock-free, facilitate automatic generation of participant-specific ("local") workflow protocols from global descriptions, and support flexible implementation of local workflows guaranteed to be compliant with the workflow protocols. The extensions with assertions and symmetric sum types support expressing *state-based (pre)conditions* and *consensual multiparty synchronisation*, which are common in complex distributed workflows.

We demonstrate the theory's applicability to *clinical practice guidelines (CPGs)* by providing a prototype implementation targeting mobile healthcare applications. It compiles declarative healthcare workflows specified in a flexible spreadsheet-formatted *process matrix* into type-checked multiparty processes. The type-checked processes are interpreted on a server communicating with generic, stateless clients running on Android tablet computers, which addresses the pervasiveness requirements common to clinical and home healthcare scenarios. A physician has, with little prior training, successfully used the prototype to design her own healthcare workflow as a process matrix, employing instantaneous test and usage feedback from the prototype.

1 Introduction

Healthcare processes are characterised by being highly mobile, collaborative, security critical, and requiring a high degree of flexibility and adaptability [3,9]. Furthermore, they typically involve complex decisions based on data collected during the process, and they are regulated, e.g. by law and clinical practice guidelines (CPGs) [25]. These characteristics make healthcare processes a particularly challenging class of case management processes [11] in need of computerised support. Their design and implementation needs to support *pervasive* execution and to be highly *trustworthy*, where formalised and verifiable process models can play

J. Weber and I. Perseil (Eds.): FHIES 2012, LNCS 7789, pp. 124–141, 2013.

a particularly important role. In the present paper we focus on how formalised models based on a compilation from a declarative process model to a new variant of multi-party session types can support pervasive execution and increase the trustworthiness. Pervasive execution is supported by automatic distribution of guideline protocols using the theory of end point projections, implemented in a prototype demonstrator allowing pervasive access to guidelines via stateless clients running on Android tablet computers. Trustworthiness is increased in two ways: 1) The declarative input format allows for specifying guidelines simply as the set of basic activities and their causal constraints instead of a procedure or flowchart. This frees the domain experts from having to "think as computers", which as stated by Parnas [20] is obviously hopeless for concurrent systems. 2) The theory of multiparty session types allows for statically guaranteeing deadlock freedom.

CPGs are descriptions of medical treatment procedures, typically maintained by professional medical associations at the national level, for specific medical disorders. CPGs can express workflows and various cooperations among healthcare processes, which are formed by the diverse collaborative patterns between multiple participants. That is, a CPG is an agreement of *global protocol* or *guideline* between distributed organisations or participants. A pattern that plays a prominent role in CPGs is what we will call *symmetric, multiparty synchronisation* where the participants collectively decide on one of the possible choices of possible next step in the protocol. Such global protocols with symmetric, multiparty synchronisations are naturally expressed in a *choreography language*, such as the WS-CDL [27] or the BPMN 2.0 [18] choreography notation exemplified in Fig. 1 in Sec. 2.

Traditionally, workflow process models and choreographies, and also CPGs, are represented as flow-graphs inspired by and based on the seminal work on the Petri Nets model [26,13], where safety and liveness properties can be verified using model checking techniques [14]. As pointed out in [9], most of this work has been focusing on centralised models and executions of the global protocols.

In the present paper we leverage the work on *session types* and *end-point projections* [8], which provides a foundation for *decentralised execution* and *verification by type checking* of protocols in general, and CPGs in particular, specified globally as choreographies. The framework of multiparty session types provides a formal choreography model language typed with *global multiparty session types* that guarantee that well-typed processes are deadlock free and can be projected to session typed end-point processes (i.e. corresponding to BPMN processes for each participant).

The work on choreographies and session types has, however, so far been focusing on process models with explicit control flow (variations of the π-calculus), which have been observed to have limitations when it comes to flexibility and adaptability [1]. As an alternative, formal declarative process notations with implicit control flow have been proposed and investigated as a means to provide more support for adaptability in case management systems in general [1,21,5,23] and health care processes in particular [6,9].

The key contributions of the present paper are to show 1) how the theory of multiparty session types [8] extended with logical predicates [4] and symmetric sum types [16] can be used to compactly represent *declarative*, distributed, and collaborative workflows, that 2) can be modelled as a global guideline by domain experts and 3) verified for deadlock-freedom statically, i.e. at compile time, using automatic code generation and type inference, and 4) interpreted in a decentralised way to provide a pervasive execution on generic tablet clients.

Concretely we show in Sec. 2 how collaborative healthcare workflows declared as *Process Matrix spreadsheets* can be automatically mapped to session typed distributed programs which are interpreted to provide a trustworthy pervasive workflow execution on Android tablet PCs. We then in Sec. 3 report on a demonstration of the prototype to a physician, who after having seen an example healthcare workflow being executed, was able to specify her own healthcare workflow declaratively as a Process Matrix spreadsheet and immediately test it on the Android tablet PCs. Finally we briefly outline in Sec. 4 the formal theory behind the approach and the properties it ensures, and describe related and future work in Sec. 5.

2   From Spreadsheets via Types to Pervasive Services

In this section we give an overview of the prototype implementation and the different technologies used by means of a simple example workflow. First, in Sec. 2.1 we describe the example workflow as a BPMN 2.0 Choreography diagram and the corresponding Process Matrix spreadsheet. We then demonstrate in Sec. 2.2 how the process matrix workflow processes can be described compactly in multiparty session types with assertions and symmetric sum types. Finally we overview the prototype implementation in Sec. 2.3.

2.1   Example Workflow as Choreography and Process Matrix

A simple CPG workflow involving three participants is described in Fig. 1 as a Choreography diagram in the Business Process Modelling Notation (BPMN) 2.0. The described workflow is activated, when a patient is admitted (indicated by the start event shown as a circle with a thin border at the left of the diagram). Then two tests, Test1 and Test2, are executed in parallel by a nurse. Note that each activity box is a *communication* between the three participants with one initiator (indicated in the white ribbon) and two receivers (indicated in the shaded ribbons). Thus, the test results are sent by the nurse to both the patient and the doctor. Each test may be repeated, as indicated by the repeating subprocess (the looping arrow), e.g. if the test failed or the result was not clear. Then, depending on the results of the tests, either the patient is discharged directly (following the bottom "ok" branch), or the doctor prescribes a drug for the patient (following the top "not ok" branch), sending the prescription to both the patient and the nurse. The workflow is ended when the patient is discharged, indicated by the end event shown as a circle with a thick border at the right

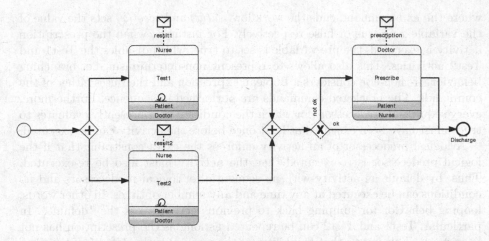

Fig. 1. Workflow as BPMN 2.0 Choreography

of the diagram. The described workflow is a standard paradigm in CPGs; that is, first a set of tests are performed and, depending on the results, either more tests are performed, the patient is discharged, or a treatment is executed. In this workflow the treatment consists of simply prescribing a drug for the patient.

For our demonstrator we do not use BPMN 2.0 choreography diagrams. Instead we use a simplified version of the declarative *Process Matrix* representation developed by our industrial partner Resultmaker (http://www.resultmaker.com/) in the TrustCare research project. The process matrix corresponding to the choreography in Fig. 1 is shown in Fig. 2 below, using three boolean data fields (pre, result1, and result2) explained below.

Id	Name	P	D	N	Seq	Log	Condition	Input	Action
1.1.1	Test1	R	R	W			¬ pre	result1	
1.1.2	Test2	R	R	W			¬ pre	result2	
1.2.1	Prescribe	R	W	R	1.1.1, 1.1.2		¬ pre ∧ ¬ (result1 ∧ result2)		set(pre)
1.3.1	Discharge	R	W	R	1.1.1, 1.1.2		(result1 ∧ result2) ∨ pre		end

Fig. 2. Example CPG workflow as Process Matrix

The process matrix has a row for each activity, and columns providing name, access control (**R**ead or **W**rite) for each participant (**P**atient, **N**urse, **D**octor), **Seq**uential predecessor relation, **Log**ical predecessor relation (not used in our simple example), Conditions, Input data, and an optional Action performed when the activity is executed. The condition field must evaluate to true for an activity to be enabled. Actions are given in a small if-then-else language:

$$Cmd ::= c \mid end,$$
$$c ::= \ set(x) \mid reset(x) \mid if \ e \ then \ c_1 \ else \ c_2 \mid \{c_1; \ldots; c_n\},$$
$$e ::= x \mid \neg \ e \mid e_1 \wedge e_2 \mid e_1 \vee e_2$$

where the *end* command ends the workflow, *set(x)* and *reset(x)* sets the value of the variable *x* to true or false respectively. For instance, when the prescription activity is executed, the pre variable is set to true, which disables the Test1 and Test2 activities. This also allows to represent non-determinism, i.e. branching behavior. If-then-else considers a Boolean expression and then uses either of the commands. The bracketed commands are performed in sequence. Furthermore, every sequential predecessor (for which the condition field presently evaluates to true) must have been executed at least once before the activity can be executed.

A logical predecessor of an activity enforces the extra constraint that if the logical predecessor is re-executed then the activity must also be re-executed. Thus, by default an activity with no sequential or logical predecessors and no conditions can be executed at any time and any number of times. In other words, looping behavior (or jumping back to previous activities) is the "default". In particular, Test1 and Test2 can be repeated as long as the prescription has not been made. This means that flexibility (of the worker) is the default; if the work flow is to be constrained, i.e. be less flexible, the constraints must be explicitly given. For instance, if tests should be allowed also after a prescription, and in that case requiring a new prescription if both tests are still not ok, one could simply change the matrix to the one given in Fig. 3.

Id	Name	P	D	N	Seq	Log	Condition	Input	Action
1.1.1	Test1	R	R	W				result1	reset(pre)
1.1.2	Test2	R	R	W				result2	reset(pre)
1.2.1	Prescribe	R	W	R		1.1.1 1.1.2	¬ pre ∧ ¬ (result1 ∧ result2)		set(pre)
1.3.1	Discharge	R	W	R	1.1.1, 1.1.2		(result1 ∧ result2) ∨ pre		end

Fig. 3. More flexible CPG with tests being logical predecessors of prescription

The same flexibility can of course be obtained using a choreography as the two notations are equally expressive, but in the process matrix notation, flexibility in execution is the default. Activities can be listed in the "normal" order, but repeated by default if necessary. Also, processes can be changed incrementally e.g. by adding rows and changing conditions. Hereto comes, that spreadsheets are familiar to many users, in particular if they have used Excel. Also, it was observed in a field study, that the tabular process descriptions actually corresponded to the paper based records used at the hospitals to keep track of the treatment [12].

2.2 Example Workflow as Multiparty Session Type

We now demonstrate how process matrix workflow processes as given above can be described compactly in multiparty session types with logical propositions as assertions and with so-called symmetric sum types.

```
μ   workflow ⟨ test1 : Bool=false , test2 : Bool=false , pre : Bool=false ,
                result1 : Bool=false , result2 : Bool=false ) .
{ Test1 [[ not pre ]]:
    3→1:1 ⟨Bool⟩ as x;              // The result of test1
    3→2:2 ⟨Bool⟩ as y [[ x=y ]];   // The result of test1
    workflow ⟨ true , test2 , pre , x , result2 ) ,
  Test2 [[ not pre ]]:
    3→1:1 ⟨Bool⟩ as x;              // The result of test2
    3→2:2 ⟨Bool⟩ as y [[ x=y ]];   // The result of test2
    workflow ⟨ test1 , true , pre , result1 , x ) ,
  Prescribe [[ test1 and test2 and not pre and not ( result1 and result2 )]]:
    2→1:3 ⟨String⟩ ;               // The prescription
    2→3:4 ⟨String⟩ ;               // The prescription
    workflow ⟨ test1 , test2 , true , result1 , result2 ) ,
  Discharge [[ test1 and test2 and (( result1 and result2 ) or pre )]]:
    end
}
```

Fig. 4. Session type representation of workflow using assertions

Multiparty session types [8] define protocols for interactions in a group of participants. They closely correspond to choreographies. In addition to defining the protocol, the theory of session types guarantees type-safety and deadlock freedom.[1] Moreover, it facilitates verifying that a collection of π-calculus processes, corresponding to BPMN processes in a collaboration diagram describing each participant, follow the specified protocol. The extension of multiparty session types with *assertions* [4] refines type signatures with logical predicates, which can be used to restrict the values that are communicated and choices that are made. We also use *symmetric sum types* [17], which are an extension of multiparty session types that can type nondeterministic choice agreed upon by multiple participants.

These three main features—multiparty, symmetric synchronisations and logical predicates—are essential for representing process matrix workflows in a direct and compact way and verifying practical use cases, not only in the context of CPGs, but also for workflows in general.

Fig. 4 specifies the workflow from Fig. 1 as a multiparty session type with symmetric sum types and assertions. The workflow is described by a *recursive type* (indicated by the initial μ sign), parameterised by a *state*: test1 and test2 describe if the respective test action has already been executed; this is needed because the test actions are sequential predecessors of the prescribe and discharge actions. The pre condition records whether the prescription activity has been executed. It is used to ensure prescription is executed only once and to block subsequent test1 and test2 actions. Finally, result1 and result2 record the results of the respective tests. The type is a symmetric sum (choice) with options specified by the underlined labels, Test1, Test2, Prescribe, and Discharge. The intuition is that all participants symmetrically agree on one of the four actions.

---

[1] This is referred to as *progress* in the theory of session types. This may be confusing, since progress is also used as synonym for liveness, i.e. that something *good* eventually happens, which is not guaranteed by the present theory of session types.

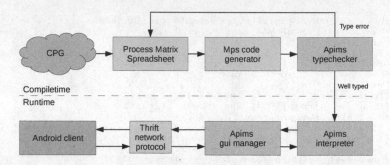

Fig. 5. Demonstrator architecture

After executing an action, the recursive type is reentered with an updated state, except if the action is Discharge, which ends the workflow. In the state where both tests have been executed, no prescription has been made yet and at least one of the test results was not ok (represented as the Boolean value false), the Prescribe, action is enabled.

The specification also describes that when Test1, is executed, the result is sent from participant 3 (the nurse) to participant 1 (the patient) and 2 (the doctor) (represented by $3 \rightarrow 1$ and $3 \rightarrow 2$).

The logical assertions are also useful for other aspects of the CPG workflows. Assertions can for example be used to enforce that doses of medicine be below a particular limit. For simplicity, this has not been included in our example, however. In the example workflow assertions are used to ensure that the same result is sent to the patient and the doctor, and control wether the medicine must be administered or the patient can be discharged directly.

2.3 Implementation

The demonstrator allows distributed execution of workflows specified by a process matrix on a server accessed by Android tablet clients. The architecture is depicted in Fig. 5. The arrow from the CPG cloud indicates that the process designer describes a workflow (e.g. a CPG) as a process matrix specification in a spreadsheet. The arrow to the mps (multi-party session types) code generator indicates that it takes the process matrix as input. In the demonstrator implementation, the process matrix is given as a comma-separated value (CSV) file produced from an off-the-shelf spreadsheet program. It enables the process matrix to be specified in a normal spreadsheet program, which provides a graphical table editor familiar to many end-users.

Code Generation. The generated mps code consists of a global multiparty session type, as exemplified in Fig. 4, representing the global workflow protocol, and the local process for each participant.

The code for the local processes contains user-interface information which, when interpreted, prompts users for information through a graphical user interface (GUI). The local process code generation, including its GUI-actions, is configurable; concretely, it is generated from descriptions written in a separate spreadsheet table.

Fig. 6 shows code for the process matrix from Fig. 2 that is very close to the actual generated code. We only show the Doctor part, as the global type is very similar to the one shown in Fig. 4. (The number 2 appearing in the code several places indicates that this is participant 2, the doctor).

```
1     link(3, wf, s, 2);
2     guivalue(3, s, 2, ".uid", "d");
3     guivalue(3, s, 2, "a121_d:title", "Prescribe");
4     ...
5     def Loop(a111: Bool, a112: Bool, a121: Bool, a131: Bool,
6              res1: Bool, res2: Bool, pre: Bool)
7              (w: wf(a111, a112, a121, a131, res1, res2, pre)@(2 of 3)) =
8     guisync(3, w, 2) {
9     a111-n 1[[not pre]]():
10        w[7] ? lungs_ok;
11        guivalue(3, w, 2, "Lungs ok?:info", lungs_ok);
12        Loop(true, a112, a121, a131,
13             (lungs_ok or ((not lungs_ok) and res1)), res2, pre)(w),
14    a112-n 1[[not pre]]():
15        w[7] ? throat_ok;
16        guivalue(3, w, 2, "Throat ok?:info", throat_ok);
17        Loop(a111, true, a121, a131, res1,
18             (throat_ok or ((not throat_ok) and res2)), pre)(w),
19    a121-d [[a111 and a112 and ((not pre) and (not (res1 and res2)))]]
20           (prescription: String = ""):
21        w[3] ! prescription;
22        w[5] ! prescription;
23        guivalue(3, w, 2, "Prescription:info", prescription);
24        guivalue(3, w, 2, ".a121_d", true);
25        Loop(a111, a112, true, a131, res1, res2, true)(w),
26    a131-d [[a111 and a112 and ((res1 and res2) or pre)]]
27           (dis_comment: String = ""):
28        end
29    }
30    in
31    Loop(false, false, false, false, false, false, false)(s)
```

Fig. 6. Mps code for Doctor participant

Corresponding to the recursion in the global session type in Fig. 4, the generated mps code consists of a single loop (line 5-31), where all actions specified in the matrix correspond to a branch (lines 9, 14, 19, 26) in a single synchronisation. Each branch is annotated with the writer of that action. In contrast to BPMN choreographies, a process matrix allows actions with more than one writer. This will be compiled to several branches in the synchronisation; e.g., if the nurse could also discharge the patient, there would be a branch a131-n .

The loop maintains a state, which includes the conditions derived from the workflow and for each action whether it has been executed. Each writer action receives inputs from the GUI (line 20) and sends them to the reader participants (lines 21, 22).

The predecessor and activity conditions are enforced using the state. Using an assertion for each branch, we can make sure a branch is only shown when its predecessors have been executed and the activity condition is true. When looping in the end of each branch, the executed state is updated in two ways:

- The executed state of the completed action, is set to true (e.g. a111 in line 12).
- The executed state of any action that has the completed action as logical predecessor is set to false.

The last part of the logic is the extra control column. The effect of the set command for action a121 can be seen in line 25, where the variable *pre* is set to true.

Apims. As part of our architecture, we have have created an ASCII syntax for the asynchronous π-calculus with multiparty sessions and symmetric synchronisation called APIMS, and implemented a type checker and an interpreter. This is to our knowledge the first prototype implementation of the π-calculus with multiparty sessions and multiparty session types. The implementation along with example programs can be found on the APIMS website [2].

The arrow connecting the mps code generation and the apims type checker in Fig. 5 shows that the mps code is type checked with the apims type checker. If the code is not well-typed it will in this case be because the workflow may deadlock, i.e. it may reach a state that is not the final state, but no activity can be executed. The example process matrices given above produce well-typed code. An innocent-looking modification such as changing the logical or ($\vee$) in the condition for the Discharge activity to a logical and ($\wedge$) would make it possible to deadlock, however: if both tests are fine (blocking the prescription), the missing prescription prevents the discharge of the patient. The static type checking thus allows the designer at compile time to catch potential deadlocks before the workflow is initiated and return to the spreadsheet and revise the specification as indicated by the arrow back to the Process Matrix Spreadsheet. [2]

If the code is well-typed, the apims interpreter in the lower right of Fig. 5 interprets the code of each participant process. It communicates with the user interfaces of the clients through a GUI manager, a separate, replaceable module that communicates with the clients and maintains a view of the global process state for each participant. In particular, each guisync term introduces a list of *choices* for each participant corresponding to enabled branches in the workflow, and each guivalue a list of *values* for each participant. The GUI manager maintains data structures for these two components, and the clients interact with the workflow by manipulating these components. The choices can be accepted by the clients, and if all parties accept a choice, execution can continue with the corresponding branch.

---

[2] However, the current implementation does not provide a very useful feedback to the non technical user.

GUI Clients. The values are used to send data to the client. Several kinds of data are transmitted: meta data, e.g. the human readable name of the different actions (as specified in the spreadsheet); value data, e.g. the data entered by the other participants; and execution data, e.g. the execution state of each action.

These data are encoded in the key-value pair of each guivalue. Note that clients are *stateless*: By keeping all data in the interpreter, clients can be changed/break down without ruining the execution.

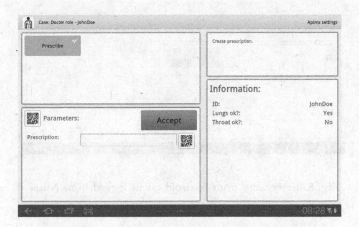

Fig. 7. Screenshot from Android client logged in as Doctor

In Fig. 6 the guivalue in line 2 assigns the Doctor role to the specific part of the code. This lets the GUI manager know which choices are assigned to which role. Fig. 7 shows a screenshot of the Android client running the example workflow in the doctor role, which can be seen at the top of the screen. The workflow is in a state where the nurse has performed both tests. The other guivalues all correspond to different parts of the screen. The guivalue in line 3 assigns the human-readable name "Prescribe" to the action a121-d . The guivalues in lines 11 and 16 are used to show the information received from the nurse (the result of the tests), which can be seen in the window to the right. Similarly the guivalue in line 23 results in the values shown on the right-hand side once the Doctor has entered those. The last guivalue in line 24 is used to pass the execution state of the action to the client. This results in a small checkmark filled with a green colour for the action, so the user knows that it has been performed. In the screenshot the execution state is false, so the checkmark is not filled, i.e. it is shown as white.

It is important to stress that every participant uses the same generic Android client. The GUI manager uses the generated code to make sure that the Android client used by the Doctor presents only the local process corresponding to the workflow relevant to the doctor, and the Android client used by the Nurse presents only the local process relevant to the Nurse. An example screenshot of the Android client running the example as the nurse role is shown in Fig. 8. It shows the workflow in a state where the nurse has performed the lung test with a negative result and still needs to perform the throat test.

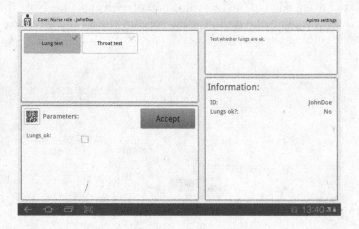

Fig. 8. Screenshot from Android client logged in as Nurse

The model-view-controller architecture of apims supports fully flexible interface design without compromising the trustworthiness of correct execution of the specified workflows. Furthermore, the communication between clients and apims is mediated through the interface definition language framework Thrift [24], which supports multiple language bindings. Altogether, this supports flexible client design for usability in a pervasive context; e.g., a simple approach to secure and efficient inputting on a tablet computer has been by using QR-codes scanned though the tablet's camera. This enables a user to scan the drug name and the dose from physical objects, minimising the amount and attendant risks of manual typing. We have only superficially touched upon the technical and usability challenges of developing user interface clients for tablet computers in comparison to conventional PC clients, however.

3   Experiment: An End-User Developed Workflow

To test the developed software, we performed a simple experiment with the help of a physician: Dorthe Furstrand Lauritzen (DFL). The motivation behind the experiment was to get first hand impressions from a domain expert, to evaluate the current implementation and set goals for future development. Although DFL is a physician and not a computer scientist, she has experience with use of IT and in particular implementation of CPGs. However, she had never seen any of the techniques used in the demonstrator before, in particular the declarative process matrix notation was completely new to her.

Id	Name	D	N	S	AN	OPN	Seq	Log	Condition
1.1.1	Nurse evaluation	R	W	R	R	R			
1.1.2	Patient History	W	R	R	R	R			
1.1.3	Extended history	W	R	R	R	R			abnorm
1.1.4	Preoperative treatment	W	R	R	R	R			cyto
1.1.5	Objective	W	R	R	R	R			
1.1.6	Extended objective	W	R	R	R	R			abnorm2
1.1.7	Ultrasound	W	R	R	R	R			
1.1.8	Formalia	W	R	R	R	R			
1.1.9	Extended formalia	W	R	R	R	R			abnorm3
1.2.0	Information for the patient	R	W	R	R	R		1.1.1 - 1.1.9	
1.2.1	Schedule for OP	R	R	W	R	W	1.2.0		

Fig. 9. End-user developed workflow (Flow)

The main component of the experiment was to put DFL in the role of the workflow designer, letting her use the spreadsheets to formalise a simple self-chosen medical workflow, which can be run on the Android tablets. There are several aspects of the experiment:

- Letting a medical professional come with a self-chosen workflow, tests the expressiveness of the system.
- Letting a new user interact with the workflow creation tool tests the usability of the tool.
- Letting a medical professional use the tool, tests the hypothesis: the domain expert can implement simple workflows, leading to a simpler and more flexible development process, e.g.
  - The domain experts might be able to make simple changes directly without involving the development team.
  - The domain experts can use simple workflows to communicate more directly and efficiently with the development team.

3.1   The Experiment

The experiment, which took a single day, was set-up as follows: DFL had access to a computer where the server, the code generator and example spreadsheets were available. To simplify the interface, all spreadsheets were placed on the desktop and batch commands performed the code generation and server start. To learn the syntax, DFL did a small exercise under instruction by one of the authors.

The workflow chosen by DFL model how a healthy woman gets an abortion; according to DFL this was "a simplification of the simplest workflow I could find".

The developed workflow is shown in Fig. 9 and Fig. 10. The roles are: Doctor (D), Nurse (N), Secretary (S), Anaesthesiologist (AN) and operation nurse (OPN).

An example screenshot from the running Android client is shown in Fig. 11.

Id	Input	Action
1.1.1	name height weight bP	
1.1.2	cave ever_birth healthy	if ! healthy then set(abnorm); if cave then set(abnorm); if ! ever_birth then set(cyto)
1.1.3	cavetx healthtx	
1.1.4	rp_cytotec	
1.1.5	gU_ia stet_c_et_p_ia uterus_retroflekteret	if ! gU_ia then set(abnorm2); if ! stet_c_et_p_ia then set(abnorm2)
1.1.6	sttx gutx	
1.1.7	fHR cRL gA	

1.1.8	clamydiatested clamydia_negative
	rhesus_negative signed_form_A
	under_18 gA_under_12
		if ! clamydiatested then set(abnorm3);
		if ! clamydia_negative then set(abnorm3);
		if rhesus_negative then set(abnorm3);
		if under_18 then set(abnorm3);
		if ! signed_form_A then reset(1.1.8);
		if ! gA_under_12 then reset(1.1.8)

1.1.9	rp_antibiotics rp_anti_D signed_form_B	
1.2.0	pt_informeret_samtykke	
1.2.1	op_tid gA_ved_op	

Fig. 10. End-user developed workflow (Data)

3.2 Evaluation

Generally the experiment turned out very successfully: DFL was easily able to use the spreadsheets to build her own workflow. The instructing author only had to take over one time to fix a problem. Even though the workflow included fairly complex logic, DFL was able to create it without any previous programming experience and despite the unwieldy syntax of the action field. The system seemed expressive enough to create the simple flow, but during the experience DFL asked for more complex logic (e.g. comparison of values) and more presentation control (e.g. grouping of values). The general usability of the tool seemed good, as DFL was able to start developing her workflow almost from the start. Of course there are several points that could be improved (most notably the action field). All in all, it is promising to let a domain expert work directly with the workflow code; maybe not for the full version, but for rapid prototyping.

4   Formal Theory

This section provides the outline of the formal theory and shows the properties which the prototype can ensure. See [16] for detailed definitions and proofs.

Once given global types as a description of global interactions among communicating processes, we can consider the following development steps for validating programs.

Step 1. A domain expert describes an intended interaction protocol as global type G with logical predicates, and checks whether is well-formed or not.

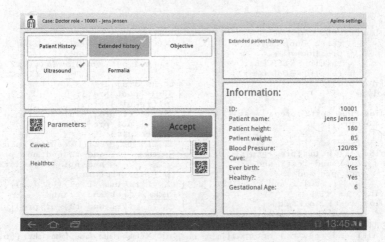

Fig. 11. Screenshot from Android client running the experiment workflow

In our implementation the global type is generated from a Process Matrix spreadsheet, by the mps code generator depicted in Fig. 5, i.e. the domain expert writes a spreadsheet instead of a global type.

Step 2. Projections of global type G (called *local types*) onto each participant are generated, either by a programmer or as in our implementation automatically.

Step 3. Program code P, one for the local behaviour of each participant p, is generated and its conformance to local type T is validated by efficient type-checking. The mps code generator in the implementation actually *creates* default implementations for each participant. A programmer can use the default implementations as starting point and then develop more refined implementations, possibly in other session typed end-point languages, while adhering to the projected local type.

When programs are executed, their interactions are guaranteed to follow the stipulated scenario without deadlocks.

Going back to the example from Sec. 2, the local type describing the behaviour of each participant can be obtained by projection (Step 2) and following this type, its process is implemented by filling input and output binding of values from the local type(Step 3). In Fig. 12 is given the local type of the patient and its behaviour described as an end-point process in the π-calculus, extended with the sync primitive. There is a clear one-to-one correspondence between type and process: for example, the recursive type μ corresponds to the recursive agent (denoted by def) and the sum type corresponds to the synchronisation (denoted by sync).

The implementation extends the π-calculus with a guisync constructor, which is the result of extending the sync for user input. Each branch has a set of typed arguments that must be given using the GUI before that choice is accepted, and the given arguments can be used by the process in that branch. In Fig. 6 guisync is seen in line 8, and the user input can be seen as "prescription" in line 20.

```
G↾1 = // Local type for Patient        P_P = // Patient
μ  workflow⟨test1:Bool=false,          ā[2..3](p,d,n).
            test2:Bool=false,          def X⟨t1:Bool,t2:Bool,pre:Bool,
            pre:Bool=false,                  r1:Bool,r2:Bool)
            result1:Bool=false,             ((p,d,n): workflow↾1⟨t1,t2,pre,
            result2:Bool=false).                              r1,r2⟩)=
{ Test1 [[not pre]]:                     sync((p,d,n),3)
  1?⟨Bool⟩ as x;                         { Test1 [[not pre]]:
  forall y[[x=y]];                         p?(result);
  workflow⟨true,test2,pre,x,result2⟩,      X⟨true,t2,pre,result,r2⟩((p,d,n)),
  Test2 [[not pre]]:                       Test2 [[not pre]]:
  1?⟨Bool⟩ as x;                           p?(result);
  forall y[[x=y]];                         X⟨t1,true,pre,r1,result⟩((p,d,n)),
    workflow⟨test1,true,pre,result1,x⟩,    Prescribe [[t1 and t2 and not pre
  Prescribe [[test1 and test2 and                      and not (r1 and r2)]]:
           not pre and                     p?(prescription);
           not (result1 and result2)]]:    X⟨t1,t2,true,r1,r2⟩((p,d,n)),
  3?⟨String⟩ as x;                         Discharge [[t1 and t2 and
  workflow⟨test1,test2,true,                          ((r1 and r2) or pre)]]}
            result1,result2⟩,            end
  Discharge [[test1 and test2 and       }
    ((result1 and result2) or pre)]]    in X⟨false,false,false,false,false⟩((p,d,n))
  end
}
```

Fig. 12. Local type and process for the patient

We then type-check processes by following the session typing rules. The typing judgement extends the original one [4] with symmetric sum types. The judgement $\Theta; \Gamma \vdash P \rhd \Delta$ states that assuming Θ the process P in the environment Γ performs exactly the session communication described in Δ. By the rules, we can verify the example is type-able, i.e. $\Theta; \Gamma \vdash (P_P \mid P_D \mid P_N) \rhd \Delta$ where P_D and P_N are the doctor and the nurse implemented similarly to P_P and | denotes parallel composition. We end this section by stating the *subject reduction theorem*, which guarantees that once the process is compiled, then there will be no type error at runtime.

Theorem 1 (Subject reduction). *If* true$; \Gamma \vdash P \rhd \emptyset$ *and* $P \rightarrow P'$, *then* true$; \Gamma \vdash P' \rhd \emptyset$.

From this theorem, we can derive many safety properties as corollaries [8, Sec. 5]. The properties which this framework guarantees include: (1) **type safety**: the lack of standard type errors in expressions; (2) **communication safety**: communication error freedom (i.e. a sending action is always matched to its corresponding receiving action at the same channel); (3) **session fidelity**: the interactions of a type-able process exactly follow the specification described by its global type; and (4) **progress**: once a communication has been established, well-typed programs will never get stuck at communication points. The formal definitions and the proofs of these properties can be found in [16,4,8].

5 Conclusions, Related and Future Work

We have successfully applied the symmetric sum types and assertion extensions of the multiparty session types to compactly specify flexible, declarative workflows with data constraints as needed for CPGs. This enables a decentralised execution automatically generated from the specification, which is guaranteed to be deadlock free by type checking and the subject reduction theorem. We provided an end-to-end, model-driven, pervasive demonstrator implementation. Finally, we reported on a successful experiment, letting a physician declaratively specify her own CPG in an off-the-shelf spreadsheet program and run it on the demonstrator.

The original implementation of the Process Matrix called *Online Consultant* by *Resultmaker* [12] is database based. This means that communication consists of the sender uploading information to the server, and all participants must query the server when using the information. Implementing the workflows based on the π-calculus and session types not only gives the Process Matrix a formal semantics, but also allows an implementation where participants communicate their data as peer-to-peer. This offers more natural and robust realisation of the workflows. It is important to point out that while the current demonstrator prototype executes all participant threads on a single, central server, there is nothing that hinders decentralised execution of such threads either on local servers or even at the clients. However, if executed (only) on a mobile client one loses the possibility to access/recover the thread if the mobile client is lost or damaged. Also, the theorem provers we have implemented (to verify assertions in the type checker) are based on the LK and CFLKF proof systems, which are not very efficient in practice. But there is an abundance of theorem provers available [22,10] which can enable both more efficient verification (in practice) and more expressive assertion languages. We can even use a resolution based theorem prover or indeed any method that can decide assertion validity, as we do not currently use the derivations for anything.

The approach in the present paper relates to work based on the Lightweight Coordination Calculus (LCC) [23,9] in being decentralised and representing clinical protocols and guidelines as message-based interaction models, which exchange information among agents distributed across different hospitals. As pointed out in [9], most other approaches ([19]) providing formal modelling, enactment and verification of CPGs have been based on centralised models and executions. While the work based on LCC focuses only on describing the individual agents, the approach based on global and local session types taken in the present paper combines the best of both worlds: the global session type corresponds to the centralised, global overview of the CPG and the local session types generated automatically from the global session type provide the individual views. Moreover, instead of relying on model checking (of the combined system of agents) the session type approach extracts the individual communication protocols which can be type-checked against an individual agent thread implemented in the π-calculus being interpreted in the current demonstrator. This also opens up possibilities for implementing local session type checking for other end-point languages, such as Java, Python, C, Ocaml, LCC and related formal notations described below.

Another related approach is the declarative Dynamic Condition Response (DCR) Graphs process model [5,15] developed in the TrustCare project.

DCR Graphs can be verified for safety and liveness properties using the SPIN model checker [15] and directly formalise the declarative process matrix model and extend it with the possibility of differentiating between may and must behaviours, that is, an activity may be possible, but not required in order to fulfil the goal of the workflow. As for the session types approach, DCR Graphs allow global descriptions from which end-point descriptions can be derived automatically and executed locally [7,6]. The distribution technique is more flexible than the one based on session types, since it is not restricted to a fixed allocation of participants in the global description. However, DCR Graphs have so far limited support for data and no facility for type and assertion checking for local agents as developed in this paper. This makes the DCR Graphs approach less flexible with respect to end point implementations which must be based on the projected DCR Graphs.

As for future work, it would indeed be interesting to explore session typed LCC, Petri Nets and DCR Graphs, which would enable to provide end-points in these languages and to include and benefit from the work on these alternative approaches. We also plan to explore an extension of session types with time deadlines and violations of such, which are crucial in order to represent real CPGs. Finally, we are planning a larger experiment with several users and CPGs in collaboration with It, Medico og Telefoni (IMT) (www.regionh.dk).

Acknowledgements. This work was funded in part by the Danish Council for Strategic Research, Grant #2106-07-0019, the IT University of Copenhagen and University of Copenhagen (the TrustCare project, www.trustcare.eu). We want to thank Dorthe Furstrand Lauritzen for participating in the experiment and for extensive feedback on the demonstrator, and the anonymous reviewers for their careful reviews and comments.

References

1. van der Aalst, W.M.P., Pesic, M., Schonenberg, H.: Declarative workflows: Balancing between flexibility and support. Computer Science - R&D 23(2), 99–113 (2009)
2. Apims project page, http://www.thelas.dk/index.php/apims
3. Bardram, J.E., Bossen, C.: Mobility work: The spatial dimension of collaboration at a hospital. CSCW 14, 131–160 (2005)
4. Bocchi, L., Honda, K., Tuosto, E., Yoshida, N.: A theory of design-by-contract for distributed multiparty interactions. In: Gastin, P., Laroussinie, F. (eds.) CONCUR 2010. LNCS, vol. 6269, pp. 162–176. Springer, Heidelberg (2010)
5. Hildebrandt, T., Mukkamala, R.R.: Declarative event-based workflow as distributed dynamic condition response graphs. In: Proceedings of PLACES 2010 (2011)
6. Hildebrandt, T., Mukkamala, R.R., Slaats, T.: Declarative modelling and safe distribution of healthcare workflows. In: Liu, Z., Wassyng, A. (eds.) FHIES 2011. LNCS, vol. 7151, pp. 39–56. Springer, Heidelberg (2012)
7. Hildebrandt, T., Mukkamala, R.R., Slaats, T.: Safe distribution of declarative processes. In: Barthe, G., Pardo, A., Schneider, G. (eds.) SEFM 2011. LNCS, vol. 7041, pp. 237–252. Springer, Heidelberg (2011)

8. Honda, K., Yoshida, N., Carbone, M.: Multiparty asynchronous session types. In: POPL 2008, pp. 273–284. ACM (2008)
9. Hu, B., Dasmahapatra, S., Robertson, D., Lewis, P.: Decentralised clinical guidelines modelling with lightweight coordination calculus. In: LBM (December 2007)
10. Kalman, J.A.: Automated reasoning with Otter. Rinton Press (2001)
11. Koehler, J., Hofstetter, J., Woodtly, R.: Capabilities and levels of maturity in IT-based case management. In: Barros, A., Gal, A., Kindler, E. (eds.) BPM 2012. LNCS, vol. 7481, pp. 49–64. Springer, Heidelberg (2012)
12. Lyng, K., Hildebrandt, T., Mukkamala, R.: From paper based clinical practice guidelines to declarative workflow management. In: ProHealth 2008 (2008)
13. MacCaull, W., Rabbi, F.: NOVA workflow: A workflow management tool targeting health services delivery. In: Liu, Z., Wassyng, A. (eds.) FHIES 2011. LNCS, vol. 7151, pp. 75–92. Springer, Heidelberg (2012)
14. Rabbi, F., Mashiyat, A.S., MacCaull, W.: Model checking workflow monitors and its application to a pain management process. In: Liu, Z., Wassyng, A. (eds.) FHIES 2011. LNCS, vol. 7151, pp. 111–128. Springer, Heidelberg (2012)
15. Mukkamala, R.R.: A Formal Model For Declarative Workflows - Dynamic Condition Response Graphs. PhD thesis, IT University of Copenhagen (2012)
16. Nielsen, L.: Regular Expressions and Multiparty Session Types with Applications to Workflow Based Verification of User Interfaces. PhD thesis, University of Copenhagen (2012)
17. Nielsen, L., Yoshida, N., Honda, K.: Multiparty symmetric sum types. In: EXPRESS 2010. EPTCS, vol. 41, pp. 121–135 (2010)
18. Object Management Group BPMN Technical Committee. Business Process Model and Notation, version 2.0. Webpage (January 2011),
    http://www.omg.org/spec/BPMN/2.0/PDF
19. Open clinical. guideline modelling methods summaries. Webpage,
    www.openclinical.org/gmmsummaries.html
20. Parnas, D.L.: Software aspects of strategic defense sytsems. Communications of the ACM 28(12), 1326–1335 (1985); Reprinted from Journal of Sigma Xi 73(5), 432-440
21. Pesic, M., van der Aalst, W.M.P.: A declarative approach for flexible business processes management. In: Eder, J., Dustdar, S. (eds.) BPM 2006 Workshops. LNCS, vol. 4103, pp. 169–180. Springer, Heidelberg (2006)
22. Riazanov, A., Voronkov, A.: The design and implementation of VAMPIRE. AI Communications 15(2, 3), 91–110 (2002)
23. Robertson, D.: A lightweight coordination calculus for agent systems. In: Leite, J., Omicini, A., Torroni, P., Yolum, P. (eds.) DALT 2004. LNCS (LNAI), vol. 3476, pp. 183–197. Springer, Heidelberg (2005)
24. Slee, M., Agarwal, A., Kwiatkowski, M.: Thrift: Scalable cross-language services implementation, http://thrift.apache.org/
25. ten Teije, A., Miksch, S., Lucas, P.: Computer-based Medical Guidelines and Protocols: A Primer and Currend Trends. Studies in Health Technology and Informatics. IOS Press (2008)
26. van der Aalst, W.M.P.: The application of Petri nets to workflow management. The Journal of Circuits, Systems and Computers 8(1), 21–66 (1998)
27. Web Services Choreography Working Group. Choreography Description Language,
    http://www.w3.org/2002/ws/chor/

A Grid Based Distributed Cooperative Environment for Health Care Research

Felipe Maia[1], Rafael Araújo[1], Luiz Carlos Muniz[1], Rayrone Zirtany[1],
Luciano Coutinho[1], Samyr Vale[1], Francisco José Silva[1], Pierpaolo Cincilla[2],
Ikram Chabbouh[2], Sébastien Monnet[2], Luciana Arantes[2], and Marc Shapiro[2]

[1] UFMA - Avenida dos Portugueses, s/n
65085-580 São Luís, MA, Brazil
{lrc,samyr,fssilva}@deinf.ufma.br
[2] UPMC - Paris, France
firstname.lastname@lip6.fr

Abstract. Providing a distributed cooperative environment is a challenging task, which requires a middleware infrastructure that provides, among others, management of distributed shared data, synchronization, consistency, recovery, security and privacy support.

In this paper, we present the ECADeG project which proposes a layered architecture for developing distributed cooperative environments running on top of a desktop grid middleware that can encompass multiple organizations. We also present a particular cooperative environment for supporting scientific research focused on the health domain. It uses the services supplied by the ECADeG architecture in order to allow researchers to share access to multiple institutions databases, visualize and analyze data by means of data mining techniques, edit research documents cooperatively, exchange information through forums and chats, etc.. Such a rich cooperative environment helps the establishment of partnerships between health care professionals and their institutions.

1 Introduction

A distributed cooperative environment provides a common user interface that enables collaborative tasks in a specific context. In such environments, many features can be provided, such as asynchronous and synchronous communication mechanisms, a repository for shared resources, or concurrent (synchronous) editing of content. Nevertheless, building a distributed cooperative environment is a challenging task, since several issues must be taken into consideration, such as managing the communication between the distributed entities, data replication, detection and resolution of update conflicts, privacy and security, provision of a WYSIWIS (What You See Is What I See) interface, and performance. As a consequence, a distributed cooperative environment is usually built on top of a middleware infrastructure that provides a set of services for hiding the complexity of the distributed environment.

The ECADeG project is a joint initiative of the Federal University of Maranhão (UFMA) Distributed Systems Laboratory, in Brazil, and the Regal Team, a joint research group of LIP6 Laboratory at University Pierre et Marie Currie (UPMC)

J. Weber and I. Perseil (Eds.): FHIES 2012, LNCS 7789, pp. 142–150, 2013.

and INRIA, France. ECADeG stands for "Enabling Collaborative Applications for Desktop Grids" and the project aims at the design and implementation of a middleware infrastructure to support the development of collaborative applications, and its evaluation through a case study in the health care domain. We established a formal partnership with the UFMA University Hospital (HU-UFMA), whose health care professionals provide the necessary medical background for the project development.

The ECADeG collaborative environment has particular concerns about security and privacy in order to deal with sensitive data such as patient and health-care information. The challenge is to follow the set of defined legal standards for medical organizations along with the specific requirements of the collaborative environment. Besides the above challenge, the platform also addresses several key challenges such as sharing data and computing resources.

This paper presents the current status of the ECADeG project. It describes the two main building blocks used as the foundation for the development of the software infrastructure proposed in ECADeG: the InteGrade, an grid middleware for desktop grids; and Telex, a middleware that facilitates the construction of collaborative applications providing optimistic sharing of documents across a network of computers. The paper also describes a preliminary view of ECADeG middleware architecture, organized as a set of layers running on top of the InteGrade grid middleware and presents the applications that comprise the cooperative environment for supporting scientific research focused at the health domain.

2   Background: InteGrade and Telex

The ECADeG middleware is being developed having as its foundation an application execution environment based on grid computing, the InteGrade middleware [1], and a middleware for supporting the development of distributed collaborative applications called Telex [2], both described in this Section.

The InteGrade project[1] is a multi-university effort to build a robust and flexible middleware for opportunistic grid computing. By leveraging the idle computing power of existing commodity workstations and connecting them to a grid infrastructure, InteGrade enables the execution of computationally-intensive parallel applications that would otherwise require expensive cluster or parallel machines.

The basic architectural unit of an InteGrade grid is a cluster, a collection of machines usually connected by a local network. Clusters can be organized in a hierarchy, enabling the construction of grids with a large number of machines.

Currently, the InteGrade middleware offers a choice of programming models for computationally intensive distributed parallel applications, MPI (Message Passing Interface), and BSP (Bulk Synchronous Parallel) applications. It also offers support for sequential and bag-of-tasks applications.

Since opportunistic grid environments are highly prone to failures, special care was taken to circumvent application execution disruptions. InteGrade provides a task-level fault tolerance mechanism based on checkpointing, which periodically saves the process' state in stable storage during the failure-free execution time [3].

---

[1] Homepage: http://www.integrade.org.br

Upon a failure, the process restarts from the latest available saved checkpoint, thereby reducing the amount of lost computation. InteGrade includes a portable application-level checkpointing mechanism for sequential, bag-of-tasks, and BSP parallel applications written in C. For MPI parallel applications, it provides a system-level checkpointing mechanism based on a coordinated protocol.

Concerning the management of application data, which includes the application binaries, input and output data, InteGrade's OppStore component provides a reliable distributed data storage using the free disk space from shared grid machines. The system is structured as a federation of clusters and is connected by a Pastry peer-to-peer network [4,5].

Telex is a generic platform that eases the development of collaborative applications. It allows application programmers to concentrate on core functionalities, by taking care of the data distribution, replication and consistency issues. Telex supports optimistic sharing over a large-scale network of computers.

Telex implements an optimistic replication approach in which updates are made locally, and are then propagated to each remote site when a communication channel is established. Update propagation is transparent to the user, and data consistency is ensured by a reconciliation protocol which runs in the background (off the critical path).

Telex is application independent although application aware. Applications need to formalize their concurrency semantics by identifying the shared data, the actions that can be made on the data and the constraints between these actions. When an end-user interacts with the application, the latter translates the operations into actions and constraints then transmits them to Telex. Based on the received local and remote actions and constraints, Telex computes sound schedules and sends them to the application to be executed. A sound schedule is a sequence of actions that satisfy the application constraints.

Schedules are computed from the Action-Constraint Graph (ACG), a replicated, dynamic graph. Actions are the nodes of the graph, and constraints the edges and arcs. A schedule is a conflict-free sub-graph.

Telex sites may generate different sound schedules from the same set of actions and constraints. A Telex module called the replica reconciler makes the sites agree on a common schedule to apply and thus achieve (eventual) mutual consistency.

ECADeG uses Telex services to manage data consistency and synchronization of distributed collaborative applications.

3   The ECADeG Project

The first aim of ECADeG project is to develop a grid-based middleware platform for the execution of distributed collaborative applications. The second one is to validate the middleware with a real distributed cooperative application, targeting the support for multi-institutional research projects in the health care domain.

The health care cooperative research environment will be based on data provided by the AGHU platform (Aplicativo de Gestão para Hospitais Universitários - Management Application for University Hospitals)[2] currently under development

---

[2] http://aghu.mec.gov.br/

by the Brazilian Ministry of Education and Culture (MEC), which implements a unified management model to be adopted by Brazilian's federal university hospitals. The AGHU database is designed to store all the data concerning patients and their care (consultations, image-based examinations, hospitalizations, surgeries, prescriptions, etc.). Some Brazilian university hospitals are already running the first available modules of AGHU on their own servers. However, each hospital runs its own copy of the AGHU platform due to the fact that each institution is administratively independent and is responsible (a trustee) for the health data that is internally generated. Therefore, the access of health data maintained by an institution by other hospitals or physicians is carefully controlled. Our middleware solution will integrate all the AGHUs installations, which would allow the university hospitals to share data and information cooperatively, as well as other computing resources, such as processor power for performing computationally intensive tasks, and specialized peripherals in a safe and controlled environment. Therefore, we will be able to provide a rich collaborative environment which helps to establish partnerships between health care professionals and their institutions.

Figure 1 shows an overview of the ECADeG architecture which consists of four main layers: Execution Environment, Core Services, Applications, and Security.

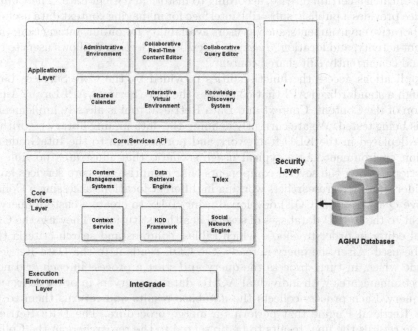

Fig. 1. ECADeG architecture

Execution Environment Layer: This layer holds the execution environment for the set of collaborative services defined by the ECADeG architecture. It is based on the InteGrade grid middlewareas described in Section 2.

Core Services Layer: The core services layer offers the set of services that supports the execution of distributed collaborative applications. The *Content Management System* provides a data space for storing any content (text, spreadsheets, data fragments retrieved from the AGHU databases, images, audio, video) shared by researchers in the context of a research project. Any stored content can be described through meta-data, whose set of attributes are defined by the application. The *Social Networking Engine* provides a complete social networking environment with bulletin boards, chats, video conferences, forums, and the tools for creating and managing users and groups. The *Data Retrieval Engine* is a tool that performs parallel data retrieval using multiple AGHU databases given an application query. It provides a SQL based API for applications and transparently manages the parallel access to multiple AGHU databases, composing a single result set as if the query was performed in a single global database. The *KDD Framework* is a component for knowledge discovery using data mining techniques to obtain relevant information from data retrieved through the Data Retrieval Engine. The framework will support classification and associations discovery tasks, since there are several possible applications of those tasks considering the medical field: (i) characterization of patients to provide further consultation, (ii) identification of successful therapies for different diseases, (iii) prediction of which patients are more likely of catch a certain disease, according to historical patient data. The *Context Service* provides a publish/subscribe interface for managing context data useful in collaborative environments, such as users availability for on-line interaction, their current activity, and location. *Telex*, as described in Section 2, allows users to create and concurrently edit shared content.

Applications access the functionalities provided by the Core Services Layer through a standardized API that comprises the Core Services API Layer. A first version of the Content, Context and Data Retrieval tool is already implemented and is being tested. We are currently defining the data mining library algorithms to be deployed in the KDD framework and porting them to the InteGrade execution environment. As a typical usage scenario that illustrates possible interactions among the several components that comprise the core services layer, consider a group or researchers working in different locations accessing a Collaborative Query Editor (CQE) developed using Telex to create a custom query to be sent to the AGHU databases of several health institutions. They use the CQE visual editor in order to choose which tables, columns and search criteria that will be used. After the query is ready, the CQE sends it to the Data Retrieval Engine which, in turn, process the query and start a process in each grid node that communicates with individual AGHU database servers in order to execute the query. Each process collects the database results and returns them to the Data Retrieval Engine that performs a merge procedure. The Data Retrieval Engine returns the final results to be presented to the researchers in the Collaborative Query Editor. They can use the Social Network engine tools to discuss and share information using chat or video-conference. If they want to process the data retrieved, e.g. for statistical analysis of the number of patients stricken by a disease in some region, the KDD framework can be used in order to run data mining algorithms to this end.

Applications Layer: In the ECADeG project we foresee the development of six main applications. The *Administrative Environment* is the tool that will be used by administrators to create, edit and delete users, define roles and enforce security policies. The *Interactive Virtual Environment* will allow users, once logged in, to interact with each other using chat, videos, forums and bulletin boards. This application uses the services provided by the Social Networking Engine and the Context Service. The *Shared Calendar* will be used for creating synchronized appointments between the platform users. Telex will be used to enforce the appointments consistency. The *Collaborative Query Editor* will create a visual query editor to the AGHU databases. Users will be able to collaboratively build queries together in real time. Telex will provide the mechanisms for maintaining the query consistency during the concurrent editing, while the Data Retrieval Engine will be used for the parallel access of the AGHU databases. The *Knowledge Discovery System* is a font-end for extracting information through data mining techniques from data retrieved using the Collaborative Query Editor. This application will be used by a KDD expert that will work together with health care researchers in order to better serve the platform users with relevant information for their research. It will use the KDD framework defined at the Core Services Layer. The *Collaborative Real-Time Content Editor* is an application that allows users to collaboratively edit shared content. In its first release, we will focus on text editing. Users will be able to concurrently edit technical reports, papers, masters and PhD thesis in real time. Again, Telex will provide the necessary tools for maintaining text consistency in the course of the concurrent editing. We already developed a first version of the ECADeG distributed collaborative environment prototype that is being validated by its final users (health care research professionals). We are also still working on the integration of the prototype functionalities with the core services layer components.

Security Layer: The security layer is transversal to all the other ECADeG layers and is based on a model that comprises a set of security policies that take into account several aspects of a collaborative environment, such as privacy and confidentiality, the organization of collaborative processes, data sharing between organizations with different administrative domains, context information and notifications of presence [6]. In addition, ECADeG security model follows the safety standards established by the Certification Manual for Electronic Registration Systems in Health (M/S-RES) [7], a document developed through a partnership between the Brazilian Society of Informatics in Health (Sociedade Brasileira de Informática na Saúde, SBIS) [3] and the Brazilian Federal Council of Medicine (Conselho Federal de Medicina, CFM)) [4]. This document describes a certification process for applications that deal with patients data, demanding that they have a complete privacy and security model, meeting the needs of users and, especially, being compliant with the legislation requirements. The ECADeG security layer includes a set of components (identity management, access control, data anonymization, auditing, and abuse report) to ensure compliance with all

---

[3] http://www.sbis.org.br/
[4] http://portal.cfm.org.br/

security policies established by its security model. The ECADeG development process also follows the steps defined in CLASP (*Comprehensive, Lightweight Application Security Process*) [8], a well defined process guided by a set of activities associated with a set software development roles that emphasizes security since the very initial phases of software development. Several security components are already implemented, such as the identity management, access control, and auditing. We are currently working on the provision of mechanisms that will allow the specification of privacy policies based on statements.

4   Related Work

Since the 80's a large amount of research has been done on distributed collaborative environments and their characteristics, as observed in [9], [10] and [11]. We can find in the literature proposals of distributed collaborative environments for various fields such as engineering ([12],[13], [14]), education ([15],[16], [17]) and health ([18], [19], [20]).By involving a large number of professionals from different areas for the design and use of collaborative environments, their development becomes complex and very dependent on the applicative domain.

A key distinctive feature of the ECADeG project is the proposal of an environment for parallel and cooperative access to databases that share a common data model and are distributed across several university hospitals. The proposals in [20] are different in the sense that they must define a WSDL[5] (Web Service Definition Language) interface with a restricted set of operations for each database where searches are made. This makes the extension of this platform more complex, and less transparent than the approach used by the middleware proposed in this article (see the Data Retrieval Engine, in the Section 3).

Similarly to [15], [16] and [18], the architecture of the ECADeG project is organized into a set of layers and modular services, including the use of computing grids. In this regard, an important difference between ECADeG and the cited works is that ECADeG is based on an opportunistic grid framework (InteGrade) that is able to run the services of ECADeG together with several classes of applications like regular, loosely coupled and tightly coupled applications. In [18] and [15], for instance, a dedicated computing grid is used only to execute processes that require intensive computation.

Compared to [18], [15], [19], [13], [12] and [20] where users have few forms of collaboration, the ECADeG project proposes a more complete set of tools to provide the users with a richer experience of collaborative working, for instance through chat rooms, video conferencing, collaborative editing of documents, file sharing, conducting search patterns using data mining algorithms, within a single workspace in order to assist them in their research.

Regarding the security aspect, the majority of the work in the literature fails to implement or suggest a full security model for the collaborative environment being proposed (with the exception of [18] that implements an initial privacy and security model based on [21]). As a consequence, there is a gap when the security

---

[5] http://www.w3.org/TR/wsdl

matters, as noted by [22]. With this concern in mind, the whole process of development, tests and validation of collaborative applications and infrastructures, in the ECADeG project, is governed by a security engineering process based on the Comprehensive Lightweight Application Security Process version 1.2 [8] (CLASP v1.2), and the set of rules present in the certification Manual for Electronic Registration Systems in Health described in the previous section. This results in a complete model of privacy and security, meeting the needs of users and, especially, which is in accordance with the requirements of Brazilian law.

5   Conclusion

This paper has described the ECADeG project, which proposes a layered architecture for developing distributed cooperative environments running on top of a desktop grid middleware. An ECADeG cooperative environment can encompass multiple organizations, sharing a variety of resources. We have also presented a particular cooperative environment for supporting scientific research focused at the health domain, which, by using the services supplied by the ECADcG architecture, provides applications for parallel access to databases of Brazilian university hospitals (using the AGHU platform), data visualization and analysis by means of data mining techniques, cooperative editing of research papers, interchange of information through forums and chats, among others. ECADeG project intends thus to provide a rich cooperative environment, which can help the partnerships between health care professionals and their institutions. By offering a virtual environment for cooperatively creating and sharing data and information, it mitigates the problem of physical distance of participants.

Acknowledgment. The authors would like to thank FAPEMA (State of Maranhão Research Agency) for the support of this work, grant INRIA-00114/11.

References

1. da Silva e Silva, F.J., Kon, F., Goldman, A., Finger, M., de Camargo, R.Y., Filho, F.C., Costa, F.M.: Application execution management on the Integrade opportunistic grid middleware. JPDC 70(5), 573–583 (2010)
2. Benmouffok, L., Busca, J.M., Marquès, J.M., Shapiro, M., Sutra, P., Tsoukala, G.: Telex: A semantic platform for cooperative application development. In: Conf. Française sur les Systemes d'Exploitation, CFSE (2009)
3. de Camargo, R.Y., Kon, F., Goldman, A.: Portable checkpointing and communication for BSP applications on dynamic heterogeneous Grid environments. In: SBAC-PAD 2005: The 17th International Symposium on Computer Architecture and High Performance Computing, Rio de Janeiro, Brazil, pp. 226–233 (October 2005)
4. de Camargo, R.Y., Kon, F.: Design and implementation of a middleware for data storage in opportunistic grids. In: CCGrid 2007: Proceedings of the 7th IEEE/ACM International Symposium on Cluster Computing and the Grid. IEEE Computer Society, Washington, DC (2007)

5. de Camargo, R.Y., Cerqueira, R., Kon, F.: Strategies for checkpoint storage on opportunistic grids. IEEE Distributed Systems Online 18(6) (September 2006)
6. Ahmed, T., Tripathi, A.R.: Security policies in distributed CSCW and workflow systems. IEEE Transactions on Systems Man and Cybernetics Part A Systems and Humans 40(6), 1220–1231 (2010)
7. Silveira, A.S., de Faria Leão, B., da Costa, C.G.A., Marques, E.P., Kiatake, L.G.G., Evangelisti, L.R., da Silva, M.L., da Costa Galvão, S., Takemae, T.T.R.: Manual de Certificação para Sistemas de Registro Eletrônico em Saúde (S-RES) (2009)
8. OWASP: CLASP v1.2 Comprehensive, Lightweight Application Security Process version 1.2. OWASP (2011)
9. Borghoff, U.M., Schlichter, J.H.: Computer-Supported Cooperative Work: Introduction to Distributed Applications. Springer, New York (2011)
10. Grudin, J.: CSCW: history and focus. IEEE Computer 27(5), 19–26 (1994)
11. Ahmed, T., Tripathi, A.R.: Security policies in distributed CSCW and workflow systems. IEEE Transactions on Systems Man and Cybernetics Part A Systems and Humans 40(6), 1220–1231 (2010)
12. Zhao, Y., Shi, X.: Collaborative computational chemical grid based on CGSP. In: Proceedings of the 2007 IFIP International Conference on Network and Parallel Computing Workshops, NPC 2007, pp. 199–202. IEEE Computer Society, Washington, DC (2007)
13. He, F., Han, S.: A method and tool for human-human interaction and instant collaboration in CSCW-based cad. Computers in Industry 57(8-9), 740–751 (2006)
14. Fan, L., Zhu, H., Bok, S.H., Kumar, A.S.: A framework for distributed collaborative engineering on grids. Computer-Aided Design 4, 353–362 (2007)
15. Jiang, J., Zhang, S., Li, Y., Shi, M.: CoFrame: a framework for CSCW applications based on grid and Web services, p. 577. IEEE (2005) Number 90412009
16. Li, Y., Yang, S., Jiang, J., Shi, M.: Build grid-enabled large-scale collaboration environment in e-learning grid. Expert Systems with Applications 31(4), 742–754 (2006)
17. Chen, J., Xiong, Z., Zhang, X.: Research on a Novel E-Learning Architecture Integrated Grid Technology, pp. 94–97. IEEE (2008)
18. Brussee, R., Porskamp, P., van den Oord, L., Rongen, E., Bloo, H., Erren, V., Schaake, L.: Integrated health log: Share multimedia patient data. In: ICME, pp. 1593–1596 (2005)
19. Lu, X.L.: System design and development for a CSCW based remote oral medical diagnosis system. In: IEEE (ed.) International Conference on Machine Learning and Cybernetics, vol. 6, pp. 3698–3703 (2005)
20. Phung, H.M., Hoang, D.B., Lawrence, E.: A novel collaborative grid framework for distributed healthcare. In: CCGRID, pp. 514–519 (2009)
21. Baumer, D., Earp, J.B., Payton, F.C.: Privacy of medical records: IT implications of HIPAA. SIGCAS Comput. Soc. 30(4), 40–47 (2000)
22. Hongxue, X., Fucai, W., Hong, Z., Mingtong, X.: A security architecture model of CSCW system. In: Management and Service Science, pp. 1–4. IEEE (2010)

Closed-Loop Modeling of Cardiac Pacemaker and Heart

Dominique Méry[1] and Neeraj Kumar Singh[2]

[1] Université de Lorraine, LORIA, BP 239, Nancy, France
Dominique.Mery@loria.fr
[2] Department of Computer Science, University of York, United Kingdom
neeraj.singh@cs.york.ac.uk

Abstract. The development of critical medical systems requires high levels of confidence in increasingly complex software systems. Formal methods have been identified as a means of contributing to assurance in this domain. We present a closed-loop modeling approach between an electrocardiography analysis based heart model and pacemaker. This stem is a step towards a modeling approach for medical systems at early stage of the system development. Implantable devices like cardiac pacemakers and implantable cardioverter-defibrillators require closed-loop modeling (integrated system and environment modeling) to qualify the certification standards. The industry has long sought such an approach to validating a system model in a virtual biological environment. This approach involves a pragmatic combination of formal specifications of the system and the biological environment to model a closed-loop system that enables verification of the correctness of the system and helps to improve the quality of the system.

Keywords: Heart Model, ECG, Cellular Automata, Event-B, Closed-loop model, Proof-based development, Refinement.

1 Introduction

In the area of medical engineering, cardiac pacemaker and implantable cardioverter-defibrillators are considered as remarkable innovations of the past century, used for saving millions of lives worldwide. The implantation rate of these devices has been increased [1–3]. Malfunctions related to the hardware and firmware are considered as a common type of defects for both pacemakers and implantable cardioverter-defibrillators [1, 4, 5]. During the 1990s, 17323 devices were explanted due to malfunction [3]. In 1996, 10% of medical device recalls were caused by software-related issues. In 2010, the Food and Drug Administration (FDA) reported 23 cases of defective devices, where some of the cases were due to software defects [1, 5–7].

Nowadays, manufacturers use standard guidelines for system development. These standards include software evaluation, which covers mainly code inspection, static analysis, module-level testing and integration testing. The purpose is to use these standards to establish *reasonable assurance of safety and effectiveness*. However, these approaches are not sufficient to check the software correctness. Testing — combined with finding bugs at the final stage of system development — is very expensive. As software plays an increasingly more important role in medical devices and in healthcare-related activities more generally, regulatory agencies such as the FDA, and certification bodies such as the FDA's Quality System Regulation and the International Standards Organization's 13485 [8, 7, 9], need effective methods for ensuring that newly developed software-based healthcare systems are *safe* and *reliable*. Regulatory agencies, in addition to the medical device manufacturers themselves, have been striving for a more rigorous engineering-based review strategy to provide this assurance [10]. Traditional methods of system development are not using formal techniques for verifying the correctness of the system requirements. An effective way of finding bugs at an early stage of the system development is practical application of formal methods. Formal methods have been successful in targeted applications of medical devices [11–14, 10, 9]. Over the past decade, there has been considerable progress in the development of formal methods for improving confidence in complex software-based systems [15, 16].

Software bugs and unexpected behaviors of the system are not easy to find from system specifications alone. To apply formal methods for verifying the specification of such complex systems is not enough. Such systems require a *closed-loop modeling approach*, where formal models of the system and an environment form a closed-loop model. The closed-loop model captures the possible behaviors of the system under environmental conditions. Such closed-loop modeling is the primary technique in system engineering and *cyber-physical* systems.

Verifying the correct behavior of a system model using an environment, is a challenging problem, where the system model and environment are both developed using identical formal notations. For example, a formal model of a cardiac pacemaker or implantable cardioverter-defibrillators requires a heart model to verify the correctness of the developed system (see Fig. 1). No tools and techniques exist for environment modeling that would enable verification of the developed system model. Most medical devices are tightly coupled with their biological environment (i.e., the heart), where these devices use sensors and actuators as interaction points. The integration of the heart and pacemaker is formally modelled and provides a good example of medical device integration [17]. In our previous work [18], we have developed a mathematical heart model. This heart model is an electro-physiological model, which models the timing and electrical conduction of the heart with both intrinsic and artificial pacing signals. In this paper, we recall the heart model for closed-loop modeling of pacemaker functionality for identifying complex behavior of the system. In the closed-loop model, the heart and pacemaker interact with each other [17]. The pacemaker responds according to the heart requirements. The heart generates all possible behaviors of the normal and abnormal conditions. The focus of this effort is three-fold: (a) we develop a mathematical heart model based on logico-mathematical theory, which provides a set of general and patient condition-specific pacemaker software requirements to ensure the safety of the patient, (b) we develop both cardiac pacemaker and heart models for closed-loop modeling, (c) we verify the closed-loop system over a variety of basic operations where the heart rate must be maintained and the atrial-ventricular synchrony must be maintained through formal proofs of the system.

The rest of this paper is organized as follows. Section 2 summarizes the construction of the heart model, which is extensively described in our previous publication [18]. Section 3 presents a closed-loop formal model of a pacemaker which interacts with the heart model. The closed-loop requirements are described in Section 4. Section 5

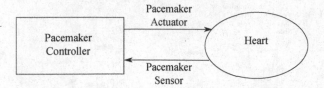

Fig. 1. Cardiac pacemaker and Heart interaction

discusses lessons learned from this experience, and Section 6 concludes the paper with some perspectives together with proposals for future work.

2   Heart Model

The heart consists of four chambers (see Fig. 2(a)): right atrium, right ventricle, left atrium and left ventricle, which contract and relax periodically. The natural heart's system requires an electrical stimulus, which is generated by the small mass of specialized tissue located in the right atrium called the sinus node. This electrical stimulus travels down through the conduction pathways and causes the heart's chambers to contract and pump out blood. Each contraction of the ventricles represents one heartbeat. The atria contract for a fraction of a second before the ventricles, so their blood empties into the ventricles, before the ventricles contract.

Fig. 2(a) presents a set of basic components and an impulse conduction path of the heart. The electrical current flows progressively in the heart muscle using special conduction cells. To model the heart system abstractly, we consider a set of landmark nodes (A, B, C, D, E, F, G, H) in the entire conduction network (see Fig. 2(b)), which provides a control behavior of the heart. These landmarks were identified in literature surveys [19–22] and extensive discussions with two experts, a cardiologist and a physiologist.

This section presents an elementary information about the heart modeling, which helps the reader to understand the modeling of the closed-loop system. A detailed description about the heart system and formalization steps are available in [18, 23]. We introduce the necessary elements using formal notations to define the heart system as follows:

Definition 1 (The Heart System). *Given a set of nodes N, a transition (conduction) t is a pair (i, j), with $i, j \in N$. A transition is denoted by $i \rightsquigarrow j$. The heart system is a tuple $HSys = (N, T, N_0, TW_{time}, CW_{speed})$ where:*

- *$N = \{$ A, B, C, D, E, F, G, H $\}$ is a finite set of landmark nodes in the conduction pathways of the heart system;*
- *$T \subseteq N \times N = \{A \mapsto B, A \mapsto C, B \mapsto D, D \mapsto E, D \mapsto F, E \mapsto G, F \mapsto H\}$ is a set of transitions to represent electrical impulse propagation between two landmark nodes;*
- *$N_0 = A$ is the initial landmark node (SA node);*

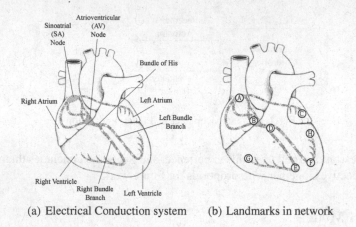

(a) Electrical Conduction system   (b) Landmarks in network

Fig. 2. The Electrical Conduction and Landmarks of the Heart System [18]

- $TW_{time} \in N \to TIME$ *is a weight function as time delay of each node, where TIME is a range of time delays;*
- $CW_{speed} \in T \to SPEED$ *is a weight function for the impulse propagation speed of each transition, where SPEED is a range of propagation speed.*

Property 1 (Impulse Propagation Time). *In the heart system, the electrical impulse originates from the SA node (node A), travels through the entire conduction network and terminates at the atrial muscle fibres (node C) and at the ends of the Purkinje fibres in both sides of the ventricular chambers (node G and node H). The impulse propagation time delay differs for each landmark node (N). The impulse propagation time is represented as the total function $TW_{time} \in N \to \mathbb{P}(0..230)$. The impulse propagation time delay for each node (N) is represented as: $TW_{time}(A) = 0..10$, $TW_{time}(B) = 50..70$, $TW_{time}(C) = 70..90$, $TW_{time}(D) = 125..160$, $TW_{time}(E) = 145..180$, $TW_{time}(F) = 145..180$, $TW_{time}(G) = 150..210$ and $TW_{time}(h) = 150..230$.*

Property 2 (Impulse Propagation Speed). *The impulse propagation speed also differs for each transition ($i \rightsquigarrow j$, where $i, j \in N$). The impulse propagation speed is represented as the total function $CW_{speed} \in T \to \mathbb{P}(5..400)$. The Impulse propagation speed for each transition is represented as: $CW_{speed}(A \mapsto B) = 30..50$, $CW_{speed}(A \mapsto C) = 30..50$, $CW_{speed}(B \mapsto D) = 100..200$, $CW_{speed}(D \mapsto E) = 100..200$, $CW_{speed}(E \mapsto G) = 300..400$ and $CW_{speed}(F \mapsto H) = 300..400$.*

Electrical activity is spontaneously generated by the SA node, which propagates through the conduction network in the entire heart system using several intermediate landmark nodes (see Fig. 2). The electrical system synchronizes the contraction between atria and ventricles. To change time intervals or conduction speeds between landmarks (see Fig. 2(b) and Fig. 2(a)) are a major cause of abnormalities in the heart system. Abnormalities in electrical signals in the heart can generate various kinds of arrhythmias. A slow conduction speed generates bradycardia and a fast conduction speed generates tachycardia. In this model, we consider the range of all possible values for conduction speeds and conduction times for each landmark node and conduction path (see Table 1). This model represents the morphological structure of the ECG signal through the conduction network (see Fig. 2(a)).

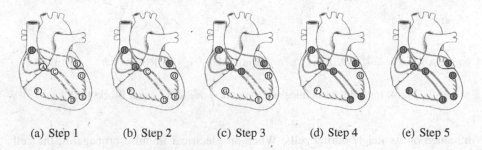

(a) Step 1   (b) Step 2   (c) Step 3   (d) Step 4   (e) Step 5

Fig. 3. Impulse Propagation through Landmark nodes [18]

Table 1. Cardiac Activation Time and Cardiac Velocity [19]

Location in the heart	Cardiac Activation Time (ms.)	Location in the heart	Conduction Velocity (cm/sec.)
SA Node (A)	0..10	A ↦ B	30..50
Left atria muscle fibers (C)	70..90	A ↦ C	30..50
AV Node (B)	50..70	B ↦ D	100..200
Bundle of His (D)	125..160	D ↦ E	100..200
Right Bundle Branch (E)	145..180	D ↦ F	100..200
Left Bundle Branch (F)	145..180	E ↦ G	300..400
Right Purkinje fibers (G)	150..210	F ↦ H	300..400
Left Purkinje fibers (H)	150..230		

Heart block is the term given to a disorder of conduction of the impulse that stimulates heart muscle contraction. The normal cardiac impulse arises in the SA node (A), situated in the right atrium, and spreads to the AV node (B), whence it is conducted by specialized tissue known as the Bundle of His (D), which divides into the left and right bundle branches in the ventricles (see Fig. 2(a)). Disturbances in conduction may appear as slow conduction, intermittent conduction failure or complete conduction failure. These three kinds of conduction failure are also known as 1st, 2nd and 3rd degree blocks. We can show these different kinds of heart block throughout the conduction network in terms of our set of landmark nodes (see Fig. 4).

A set of spatially distributed cells form a Cellular Automata (CA) model, which contains a uniform connection pattern among neighbouring cells and local computation laws. CA are discrete dynamic systems corresponding to space and time, which provide uniform properties for state transitions and interconnection patterns. The cardiac muscle cells of the heart are presented in the following states: *Active*, *Passive* or *Refractory*. Initially, all cells are *Passive*, where each cell is discharged electrically and has no

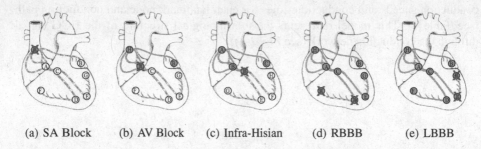

(a) SA Block   (b) AV Block   (c) Infra-Hisian   (d) RBBB   (e) LBBB

Fig. 4. Impairments in Impulse Propagation due to the Heart Blocks [18]

influence on its neighbouring cells. When an electrical impulse propagates, the cell becomes charged and eventually activated (*Active* state). The *Active* cell transmits an electrical impulse to its neighbour cells. The electrical impulse is propagated to all the cells in the heart muscle. After activation, the cell becomes discharged and enters the *Refractory* state within which the cell can not be reactivated. After a time, the cell changes its state to the *Passive* state to await the next impulse.

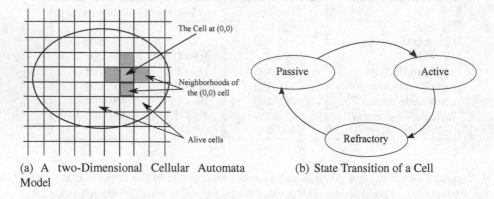

(a) A two-Dimensional Cellular Automata Model   (b) State Transition of a Cell

Fig. 5. Two-Dimensional Cellular Automata and State Transition Model [18]

3   Closed-Loop Model of Heart and Cardiac Pacemaker

This section describes a closed-loop formal model of a cardiac pacemaker and of the heart system, where the cardiac pacemaker responses according to the functional behavior of the heart [18, 23]. The main objective of this model is to verify the complex properties of the cardiac pacemaker under the virtual environment. Fig. 1 represents a block diagram of the cardiac pacemaker and of the heart system, where the cardiac pacemaker responses, when it senses intrinsic activities from the heart. In this system specification, the heart model simulates the functional behavior of the normal and abnormal heart rate. The heart model activities are always monitored by the cardiac pacemaker and it responses according to the user needs.

In our previous work, we have already developed the formal model of the cardiac pacemaker [24] and of the heart system [18]. This paper presents a closed-loop model of the cardiac pacemaker, where the heart is used as an environment. For developing this closed-loop model, we borrow formal specifications from the previously developed and verified formal models of the cardiac pacemaker [24] and heart system [18]. However, to develop the closed-loop model, we have done substantial changes in the existing models to specify the desired behavior of the system. Moreover, we develop the whole system from scratch using progressive refinements. Each refinement level introduces both cardiac pacemaker and heart system behaviors. To check the correctness of the closed-loop system, we have introduced safety properties using invariants, and discharged all the generated proof obligations at each refinement level. Due to space limitations, the following section formalizes the closed-loop system abstractly.

3.1   The Context and Initial Model

To formalize the heart behavior, we capture the electrical features. We identify a set of landmark nodes from the conduction network (see Fig. 2(a)) of the heart. These landmark nodes are also known as the electrical impulse propagation nodes *ConductionNode*, which enable expression of the normal and abnormal behaviors of the heart system. We find the direct connections among the impulse propagation nodes, which constitute the impulse propagation path. The impulse propagation time and the impulse propagation velocity for each pair of nodes vary due to different types of muscles in the heart. To formalize the heart system, we define three constants impulse propagation time *ConductionTime*, impulse propagation path *ConductionPath* and impulse propagation velocity *ConductionSpeed*. All these constants are initial components, which are defined through a set of axioms ($axm1$-$axm4$). To formalize the cardiac pacemaker, we define a set of constants ($LRL, URL, ARP, VRP, PVARP$ etc.), which express timing intervals. These timing intervals are used as a set of configuration parameters. To model a boolean behavior of the sensor and actuator, we define an enumerated set *status*. Axioms for the cardiac pacemaker are defined by $axm5$ and $axm6$. All these constants and axioms have been extracted from the definitions (see Section 2) and technical specification [25], that are validated by the cardiologist and the physiologist.

$axm1 : partition(ConductionNode, \{A\}, \{B\}, \{C\}, \{D\}, \{E\}, \{F\}, \{G\}, \{H\})$
$axm2 : ConductionTime \in ConductionNode \rightarrow \mathbb{P}(0 .. 230)$
$axm3 : ConductionPath \subseteq ConductionNode \times ConductionNode$
$axm4 : ConductionSpeed \in ConductionPath \rightarrow \mathbb{P}(5 .. 400)$
$axm5 : LRL \in 30 .. 175 \wedge URL \in 50 .. 175 \wedge PVARP \in 150 .. 500$
$axm6 : ARP \in 150 .. 500 \wedge VRP \in 150 .. 500 \wedge status = \{ON, OFF\}$

To define an abstract model of the closed-loop system, we develop the combined model of the cardiac pacemaker and of the heart, where the cardiac pacemaker acts according to the heart behavior. The environment model of the heart behaves according to the observations of the impulse propagation in the conduction nodes. We define a set of variables to model the heart and pacemaker models, where four variables (*ConductionNodeState*, *CConductionTime*, *CConductionSpeed* and *HeartState*) are used to model the heart behavior, and six variables(*PM_Actuator_A*,*PM_Actuator_V*, *PM_Sensor_A*, *PM − _Sensor_V*, *Pace_Int* and *sp*) are used to express the cardiac pacemaker behavior. All these variables are defined using a list of invariants (*inv1-inv7*). The cardiac pacemaker variables are introduced for modeling actuators, sensors and timing intervals. A list of invariants (*inv8*,*inv9* and *inv10*) presents safety properties. The invariant *inv8* states that, when the clock counter *sp* is less than VRP and atrioventricular (AV) counter state *AV_Count_State* is FALSE, then the pacemaker's actuators and sensors of both chambers are OFF. Similarly, the next invariants (*inv9* and *inv10*) represent the required properties of ON state of the pacemaker's actuators in both chambers.

$$inv1 : ConductionNodeState \in ConductionNode \rightarrow BOOL$$
$$inv2 : CConductionTime \in ConductionNode \rightarrow 0 .. 300$$
$$inv3 : CConductionSpeed \in ConductionPath \rightarrow 0 .. 500$$
$$inv4 : HeartState \in BOOL$$
$$inv5 : PM\_Actuator\_A \in status \land PM\_Actuator\_V \in status$$
$$inv6 : PM\_Sensor\_A \in status \land PM\_Sensor\_V \in status$$
$$inv7 : Pace\_Int \in URI .. LRI \land sp \in 1 .. Pace\_Int$$
$$inv8 : sp < VRP \land AV\_Count\_STATE = FALSE \Rightarrow$$
$$PM\_Actuator\_V = OFF \land PM\_Sensor\_A = OFF \land$$
$$PM\_Sensor\_V = OFF \land PM\_Actuator\_A = OFF$$
$$inv9 : PM\_Actuator\_V = ON \Rightarrow sp = Pace\_Int \lor (sp < Pace\_Int \land$$
$$AV\_Count > V\_Blank \land AV\_Count \geq FixedAV)$$
$$inv10 : PM\_Actuator\_A = ON \Rightarrow (sp \geq Pace\_Int - FixedAV)$$

The abstract specification of the closed-loop model contains several events related to the cardiac pacemaker and to the heart system. There are many events, namely *HeartOK* to represent a normal state of the heart, *HeartKO* to express an abnormal state of the heart, *HeartConduction* to trace the current updated value of each landmark node in the conduction network, *Actuator_ON_V*, *Actuator_OFF_V*, *Actuator_ON_A* and *Actuator_OFF_A* to represent ON and OFF states of the pacemaker's actuators for both chambers, *Sensor_ON_A*, *Sensor_OFF_A*, *Sensor_ON_V*, and *Sensor_OFF_V* to represent ON and OFF states of the pacemaker's sensors for both chambers, and *tic* to represent clock counter. Due to space limitations, we describe few events in detail.

The event *HeartOK* expresses desired behavior of the normal heart, where a set of guards formulates the required conditions. The first guard (*grd1*) states that all the landmark nodes must be visited for one cycle during impulse propagation using conduction network. The second guard specifies that the current impulse propagation time for each landmark node should be ranged in the pre-specified ranges (*Property 1*). Similarly, the last guard states that the current impulse propagation velocity of each path should range between pre-defined impulse propagation velocities (*Property 2*). The action predicate (*act1*) denotes the normal state of the heart, when these guards are satisfied.

```
EVENT HeartOK
  WHEN
    grd1 : ∀i·i ∈ ConductionNode ⇒ ConductionNodeState(i) = TRUE
    grd2 : ∀i·i ∈ ConductionNode ⇒ CConductionTime(i) ∈ ConductionTime(i)
               ⎛ i ↦ j ∈ ConductionPath                                      ⎞
    grd3 : ∀i, j· ⎜ ⇒                                                         ⎟
               ⎝ CConductionSpeed(i ↦ j) ∈ ConductionSpeed(i ↦ j)            ⎠
  THEN
    act1 : HeartState := TRUE
  END
```

In the two electrodes pacemaker, we use two sensors and two actuators for capturing the required behavior of the cardiac pacemaker. In this section, we show only actuator and sensor events of the ventricle chamber. Moreover, other events related to the sensor and actuator of the atrial chamber are identical. Events $Actuator\_ON\_V$ and $Sensor\_ON\_V$ are excerpt from the abstract model to describe ON state of the actuator and sensor of the cardiac pacemaker. A list of guards of both events enables to set ON state of both actuator and sensor, allowing to pace and to sense in the ventricular chamber under the desired conditions using real-time constraints. A detailed formalization of the other events related to the cardiac pacemaker are described in [24, 26].

```
EVENT Actuator_ON_V
  WHEN
    grd1 : PM_Actuator_V = OFF
    grd2 : (sp = Pace_Int)∨
              (sp < Pace_Int∧
               AV_Count > V_Blank ∧
               AV_Count ≥ FixedAV)
    grd3 : sp ≥ VRP ∧ sp ≥ PVARP
              ∧sp ≥ URI
  THEN
    act1 : PM_Actuator_V := ON
    act2 : last_sp := sp
  END
```

```
EVENT Sensor_ON_V
  WHEN
    grd1 : PM_Sensor_V = OFF
    grd2 : (sp ≥ VRP ∧ sp < Pace_Int − FixedAV∧
            PM_Sensor_A = ON)
            ∨
            (sp ≥ Pace_Int − FixedAV ∧
             AV_Count_STATE = TRUE)
    grd3 : PM_Actuator_A = OFF
  THEN
    act1 : PM_Sensor_V := ON
  END
```

In our previous models [18, 23, 24, 26]. of the cardiac pacemaker and of the heart system, we use the tic event to model a clock, separately. However, in the closed-loop model, we use a *single* event tic to specify a common clock for both cardiac pacemaker and heart environment models. The event tic models the clock behavior, where time is progressively increased using the current clock counter sp. It controls the time line of pacing and sensing events. A guard ($grd1$) of this event provides the required conditions to increase the clock counter sp by 1 (ms.).

```
EVENT tic
  WHEN
    grd1 : (sp < VRP)
            ∨
            (sp ≥ VRP ∧ sp < Pace_Int − FixedAV ∧
             PM_Sensor_A = ON ∧ PM_Sensor_V = ON)
  THEN
    act1 : sp := sp + 1
  END
```

3.2   Chain of Refinements

So far, we have described our abstract model of the closed-loop model. Each refinement level is used to introduce a new set of functional properties for modeling the normal and abnormal behaviors of the heart and of the pacemaker. Rather than presenting a chain of refinement stages in detail, we give an overview of the remaining refinement stages, sufficient to explain the rationale of each refinement stage in formalizing the system. For more detailed information, see in [23, 24, 18, 26].

Refinement 1: Introducing *threshold* in Cardiac Pacemaker and Impulse Propagation in the Heart System. This refinement step is known as a conduction model, which introduces the impulse propagation in the conduction network of the heart. The impulse propagation originates from the SA node and passes through all the landmark nodes and reaches at the Purkinje fibers of the ventricles. We formalize the conduction model by the introduction of a set of events, which supports piecewise development of the impulse propagation. The electrical impulse passes through several intermediate landmark nodes and finally sinks to the terminal nodes (C, G, H). The conduction model uses the clock counter to model the real-time system to satisfy the required temporal properties for the impulse propagation. A set of new events simulates the desired behavior of the impulse propagation into the heart conduction network, where each new refined event formalizes impulse flow between two landmark nodes; for instance, the electrical impulse moves from SA node (A) to AV node (B).

In the refinement of the closed-loop system, the cardiac pacemaker development introduces sensors behavior for both atrial and ventricular chambers, which models the sensing activities using some standard threshold values. The threshold values are different for both atrial and ventricle chambers. The heart conduction behavior is continuously monitored by the cardiac pacemaker model. The monitored value is compared with the standard threshold value under the required timing intervals to allow or inhibit to pace into the heart chamber for controlling the desired behaviors of the heart.

Refinement 2: Introduction of Hysteresis for Cardiac Pacemaker Model and Perturbation of the Conduction for the Heart Model. This refinement step introduces an abnormal behavior in the closed-loop model through introduction of the blocking activities, and *hysteresis* operating mode in the cardiac pacemaker model. The blocking behavior in the heart network is known as perturbation model, which specifies perturbations in the heart conduction system and helps to discover exact blocks into the heart conduction network. We introduce a set of events through progressive refinement to simulate the desired blocking behavior. The blocking behavior generates troubles into electrical impulse propagation. Different types of heart blocks are presented through the partition of the landmark nodes in the conduction network.

The cardiac pacemaker model uses the refinement to introduce a new feature related to the operating modes. This new feature is known as the *hysteresis* operating mode, which prevents the constant pacing and allows a patient to have his/her own underlying rhythm as much as possible. The *hysteresis* is a programmed feature whereby the pacemaker paces at a faster rate than the sensing rate. This refinement introduces a new event, which allows to set *hysteresis* mode, and the cardiac pacemaker operates according to the desired rate.

Refinement 3: Introduction of Rate Modulation for the Cardiac Pacemaker Model and a Cellular Model for the Heart System. This is the final refinement of the closed-loop system, which introduces the cellular level modeling for the heart system and the rate modulation for the cardiac pacemaker. The final refinement of the heart system provides a simulation model, which introduces the impulse propagation at the cellular level using cellular automata. The electrical impulse propagates at the cells level. A set of constants and mathematical properties is introduced using axioms, and a set of events is used to formalize the desired behaviors of the heart using cellular automata, which are described in [18].

In the final model of the cardiac pacemaker, we describe a rate adapting pacing tech- nique. The rate adapting pacing technique gives freedom to select automatically desired pacing rate according to the physiological needs. Automatic selection of the desired pacing rate helps to increase or to decrease the pacing rate and assists a patient for controlling the heart rate according to the different day to day activities. In the rate modulation mode, the pacemaker operates faster than the lower rate, but no more than the upper sensor rate limit, when it determines then the heart rate needs to increase. For instance, when a patient does an exercise, the heart rate cannot increase automatically to fulfill the required pumping rate. The rate modulation sensor is used to determine the maximum exertion performed by the patient. This increased pacing rate refers to the *sensor indicated rate*. Reducing the physical activities helps to progressively decrease the pacing rate down to the lower rate. A set of new refined events models increasing and decreasing pacing rate of the cardiac pacemaker.

3.3   Proof Statistics

Table 2 contains the proof statistics of the development of the closed-loop model of the cardiac pacemaker with the heart system. These statistics measure the size of the model, the proof obligations (POs) generated and discharged by the RODIN prover and those that are interactively proved. The complete development of the closed-loop model model results in 3049 (100%) POs, within which 2147 (70%) are proved automatically by the RODIN tool.

Table 2. Proof Statistics

Model	Total number of POs	Automatic Proof	Interactive Proof
Closed-loop model of One-electrode pacemaker			
Abstract Model	304	258(85%)	46(15%)
First Refinement	1015	730(72%)	285(28%)
Second Refinement	72	8(11%)	64(89%)
Third Refinement	153	79(52%)	74(48%)
Closed-loop model of Two-electrode pacemaker			
Abstract Model	291	244(84%)	47(16%)
First Refinement	1039	766(74%)	273(26%)
Second Refinement	53	2(4%)	51(96%)
Third Refinement	122	60(49%)	62(51%)
Total	3049	2147(70%)	902(30%)

The remaining 902 (30%) POs are proved interactively using the RODIN tool. In- tegration of the heart model and the cardiac pacemaker model generates lots of extra POs. The main reason of these new POs is to use shared variables in both models to link between the heart and pacemaker models. A set of invariants corresponding to the shared variables generates new POs. For example, the current clock counter variable (sp) is shared, which has been used in events of the heart and pacemaker models. The com- bined invariants of the heart and pacemaker models generates new POs corresponding to the current clock counter variable (sp). The whole system represents functional prop- erties of the cardiac pacemaker operating modes under the biological environment in the heart. The heart model represents normal and abnormal states of the heart, which is estimated by the physiological analysis. To guarantee the correctness of these functional behaviors, we have established various invariants in the incremental refinements.

Model checking [27] is a complementary technique for validation and verification of a formal specification. The model checker investigates expected system behaviors under the required safety properties and confirms the correctness of the closed-loop system. The use of model checker helps to discover some unexpected behaviors, and assists to verify all the operating modes of the cardiac pacemaker in the heart environment model. A tool ProB [28] is used to animate the closed-loop model and able to prove the absence of errors [26].

4 Closed-Loop Modeling Requirements

This section presents a set of requirements for modeling the closed-loop system in order to guarantee the safety properties [2]. These requirements are useful for verifying the closed-loop system.

4.1 Patient Safety in Closed-Loop

The closed-loop system must meet a set of requirements related to the physiological needs. The heart's state indicates the patient's condition, which presents conditional properties. In the closed-loop system, the heart states are connected to the heart model parameters, which are not affected by pacemaker therapy. The integration of the heart model and pacemaker model allows us to evaluate whether the pacemaker provides an appropriate therapy for any arrhythmias.

4.2 Behavioral Requirements

The closed-loop system exposes several conditions for both normal and abnormal heart functionalities, which are represented through node automata (Fig. 2(b)) using ranges of impulse propagation speed and impulse propagation time. The condition is a boolean value for meaning whether the heart state is true. The cardiac pacemaker presents pacing and sensing activities under specified conditions. Some behavioral requirements are given as follows: 1) Atrial and ventricular paces should not occur during atrial and ventricular refractory period, respectively. This requirement is an important safety property, which is verified in the closed-loop model. Any pacing during the refractory period creates derangements in timing for the atria and ventricles. 2) Intrinsic activities of the atria and ventricles should be sensed by different leads. The intrinsic activities are essential input for the pacemaker. The pacemaker should ensure that the intrinsic activities are sensed accurately. 3) Natural pacing in the atria and ventricles, and artificial pacing and sensing activities of the pacemaker must be coordinated to ensure efficient pumping for maintaining the heart rhythm.

4.3 Clinical Requirements with Closed-Loop

Clinical requirements depend on the patient needs such as normal sinus rhythm, bradycardia, heart block and tachycardia. These requirements are common critical conditions, which can vary between patients because of different physiological needs.

In this paper, the heart model is as abstract as possible to capture all possible scenarios of the heart, which is completely based on the conduction speed and conduction time. Whenever these two parameters change or lie out of the range, then the ECG signal deforms and we cannot obtain the desired ECG signal, which represents an abnormal heart state. Moreover, we have introduced heart blocking behavior using stepwise refinement. Rather then considering any particular behavior of the heart, we have abstractly formalized the heart. For instance, we have not processed any special treatment in our model to capture the retrograde conduction (travel backwards). We have considered the perfect heart condition (see HeartOK, where we have only a forward conduction network). The retrograde conduction results in many different symptoms, primarily those symptoms resulting from the delayed, non-physiologic timing of atrial contraction in relation to ventricular contraction. According to our model, if the retrograde conduction affects the timing cycle or conduction speed, then the heart presents an abnormal state. The normal state of the closed-loop model is presented according to the timing and speed of the conduction requirements. In case of abnormal state of the heart, the cardiac pacemaker paces and senses according to the patient's needs. In this closed-loop system, the cardiac pacemaker can take effect, when the heart presents an abnormal state, which helps to maintain the patient heart rhythm. We have considered heart state (OK or KO) for each cycle. If the cycle has any abnormality, the heart will be in abnormal state and the pacemaker takes over to maintain the heart rhythm. In addition, this closed-loop model helps to identify the pacemaker requirements according to the heart behavior.

5   Discussion

This paper presents an approach for modeling the closed-loop system. The prime objective of this approach is to provide a new modeling technique, which helps to combine the formal models of a critical system and related environment. For example, the cardiac pacemaker operates in the biological heart system. The closed-loop modeling is an effective approach, which guarantees the correctness of the operating behavior of the critical system. Moreover, this approach provides a viable mechanism for obtaining the certification standards for the system development. To build a closed-loop model using both environment and device modeling, is considered as a standard approach for validation, given that designing an environment model is a challenging problem in the real world. Industry has long sought such an approach to validating system models in a biological environment. We have proposed the closed-loop modeling approach, which is based on our previous research related to the cardiac pacemaker [24] and to the heart model [18].

A Virtual Heart Model (VHM) based on Simulink has been developed by Jiang et al. [2], which can be used for testing a pacemaker. However, a major constraint of their approach is that the VHM and pacemaker both use the Simulink, which is not based on any formal technique such as a theorem prover or model checker. Therefore, it is not feasible to integrate their VHM with any formal methods based cardiac pacemaker model in order to build a closed-loop system. A wide range of work related to the formal verification of the pacemaker has been presented [24, 29, 30], but none of these has used the heart environment model for verification purpose. We have proposed modeling the heart in an abstract way to simulate the desired behavior of the heart system whilst avoiding the complexity, which is based on logico-mathematical theory [18]. Our proposed approach for modeling the closed-loop system of the heart and pacemaker is better than existing modeling approach. The closed-loop model of the heart and pacemaker is developed using a refinement-based approach and has been used to verify the system properties under patient conditions.

6   Conclusion

We present a method for modeling pacemakers within the closed-loop context of a heart model. The heart model is based on logico-mathematical theory and is the first computational model [18] that considers the heart as an electrical conduction system. Given that a cardiac pacemaker interacts with the heart exactly at this level (i.e., electrical impulses), this model is a very promising *environmental model* to be used in parallel with a pacemaker model to form a closed-loop system. It therefore has an immediate use in *the grand challenges in formal methods* where an industrial pacemaker specification has been elected as a benchmark. To model the closed-loop system of the heart and cardiac pacemaker, we have used the Event-B modeling language[31, 15]. Our approach involves formalizing and reasoning about behavior of a cardiac pacemaker under normal and abnormal heart conditions. A set of general and patient condition-specific temporal requirements is specified for the closed-loop system. Based on these requirements, we have presented an interactive and physiologically relevant closed-loop model for verifying basic and complex operations of the cardiac pacemaker. With the use of model checkers, we demonstrate that the proposed system is capable of testing common and complex heart conditions across a variety of pacemaker modes. This system is a step towards a modeling approach for medical cyber-physical systems with the patient-in-the-loop. The main objectives of the proposed idea are as follows:

- To meet the certification standards
- To verify a critical system like a cardiac pacemaker or implantable cardioverter-defibrillators in a patient model (using a formal representation)
- To analyse the interaction between the heart model and a cardiac pacemaker or implantable cardioverter-defibrillators.

Applying the closed-loop approach for developing the cardiac pacemaker has many benefits, including the exposure of errors which might have not been detected without the environment model. A list of guidlines proposed by regulatory standards (NITRD, IEEE, and IEC/ISO) allows adoption of the closed-loop modeling using formal techniques to establish mechanisms for verifying the specification against the user requirements and certification standards, and to ensure that designs and programs satisfy their requirements specifications.

   We have outlined how an incremental refinement approach to the closed-loop model of the heart and pacemaker system enables a high degree of automatic proof using the RODIN tool. Our various developments reflect not only many facets of the problem, but also the learning process involved in understanding the problem and its ultimate possible solutions. The consistency of our specification has been checked through reasoning, and validation experiments were performed using the ProB model checker with respect to safety conditions. At each stage of the refinement, we have introduced a new behavior for the system and proved its consistency and performed refinement checking. We have introduced more general invariants at the refinement level, showing that the initialization of the whole system is valid. Finally, we have verified the correctness of the exact behavior of our closed-loop system with the help of physiology and cardiology experts.

As a part of our future efforts we plan to generate the automatic test cases from this closed-loop model, permitting system testing. In addition, it would be beneficial to consider a more complex pacemaker model such as the three electrodes pacemaker. Finally, as future work we plan to implement the developed closed-loop formal model. With this approach, our goal is to generate this closed-loop model, moving from a formal model to a Simulink model, which is the most common approach for realizing a real-time system. The final implemented system will comply with developed closed-loop formal models.

Acknowledgement. We are grateful to cardiologist experts Prof. Yves Juillière (MD, Cardiology) and Dr. Frédérique Claudot (PhD) and biomedical experts Dr. Didier Fass (PhD) of the Université de Lorraine, who shared their experience with us. We are thankful to the anonymous reviewers for their helpful and detailed comments.

References

1. Sandler, K., Ohrstrom, L., Moy, L., McVay, R.: Killed by code: Software transparency in implantable medical devices (2010)
2. Jiang, Z., Pajic, M., Mangharam, R.: Model-based closed-loop testing of implantable pacemakers. In: 2011 IEEE/ACM International Conference on Cyber-Physical Systems (ICCPS), pp. 131–140 (April 2011)
3. Maisel, W.H., Sweeney, M.O., Stevenson, W.G., Ellison, K.E., Epstein, L.M.: Recalls and safety alerts involving pacemakers and implantable cardioverter-defibrillator generators. JAMA: The Journal of the American Medical Association 286(7), 793–799 (2001)
4. US FDA Center for Devices and Radiological Health: Medical devices; current good manufacturing practice (cgmp) final rule; quality system regulation (1996)
5. US FDA Center for Devices and Radiological Health: Guidance for the content of premarket submissions for software contained in medical devices (May 2005)
6. Center for Devices and Radiological Health: Safety of Marketed Med. Devices, FDA (2006)
7. A Reseach and Development Needs Report by NITRD: High-Confidence Medical Devices : Cyber-Physical Systems for 21st Century Health Care,
   http://www.nitrd.gov/About/MedDevice-FINAL1-web.pdf
8. Keatley, K.L.: A review of the fda draft guidance document for software validation: guidance for industry. Qual. Assur. 7(1), 49–55 (1999)
9. Lee, I., Pappas, G.J., Cleaveland, R., Hatcliff, J., Krogh, B.H., Lee, P., Rubin, H., Sha, L.: High-confidence medical device software and systems. Computer 39(4), 33–38 (2006)
10. Méry, D., Singh, N.K.: Trustable formal specification for software certification. In: Margaria, T., Steffen, B. (eds.) ISoLA 2010, Part II. LNCS, vol. 6416, pp. 312–326. Springer, Heidelberg (2010)
11. Bowen, J., Stavridou, V.: Safety-critical systems, formal methods and standards. Software Engineering Journal 8(4), 189–209 (1993)
12. Jetley, R.P., Carlos, C., Iyer, S.P.: A case study on applying formal methods to medical devices: computer-aided resuscitation algorithm. International Journal on Software Tools for Technology Transfer 5(4), 320–330 (2004)

13. Jetley, R., Purushothaman Iyer, S., Jones, P.: A formal methods approach to medical device review. Computer 39(4), 61–67 (2006)
14. Méry, D., Singh, N.K.: Real-time animation for formal specification. In: Aiguier, M., Bretaudeau, F., Krob, D. (eds.) Complex Systems Design & Management, pp. 49–60. Springer, Heidelberg (2010)
15. Abrial, J.R.: Modeling in Event-B: System and Software Engineering. Cambridge University Press (2010)
16. Fitzgerald, J.S.: The typed logic of partial functions and the vienna development method. In: Bjørner, D., Henson, M.C. (eds.) Logics of Specification Languages. Monographs in Theoretical Computer Science. An EATCS Series, pp. 453–487. Springer, Heidelberg (2008)
17. Lieber, R., Fass, D.: Human systems integration design: Which generalized rationale? In: Kurosu, M. (ed.) Human Centered Design, HCII 2011. LNCS, vol. 6776, pp. 101–109. Springer, Heidelberg (2011)
18. Méry, D., Singh, N.K.: Formalization of heart models based on the conduction of electrical impulses and cellular automata. In: Liu, Z., Wassyng, A. (eds.) FHIES 2011. LNCS, vol. 7151, pp. 140–159. Springer, Heidelberg (2012)
19. Malmivuo, J., Plonsey, R.: Bioelectromagnetism: Principles and Applications of Bioelectric and Biomagnetic Fields, 1st edn. Oxford University Press, USA (1995) ISBN 0-19-505823-2
20. Khan, M.G.: Rapid ECG Interpretation. Humana Press (2008)
21. Bayes de Luna, A., Batcharov, V.N., Malik, M.: The morphology of the Electrocardiogram. In: John Camm, A., Lascher, T.F., Serruys, P.W. (eds.) The ESC Textbook of Cardiovascular Medicine. Blackwell Publishing Ltd. (2006)
22. Artigou, J.Y., Monsuez, J.J., Société française de cardiologie: Cardiologie et maladies vasculaires. Elsevier Masson (2006)
23. Méry, D., Singh, N.K.: Technical Report on Formalisation of the Heart using Analysis of Conduction Time and Velocity of the Electrocardiography and Cellular-Automata. Technical report, LORIA UMR7503 - Université de Lorraine (May 2011)
24. Méry, D., Singh, N.K.: Functional behavior of a cardiac pacing system. International Journal of Discrete Event Control Systems 1(2), 129–149 (2011)
25. Boston Scientific: Pacemaker system specification, Technical report (2007), http://www.cas.mcmaster.ca/sqrl/SQRLDocuments/PACEMAKER.pdf
26. Singh, N.K.: Reliability and Safety of Critical Device Software Systems. PhD in Computer Science, Université Henri Poincaré - Nancy 1, France (November 2011), http://www.scd.uhp-nancy.fr/docnum/SCD_T_2011_0129_SINGH.pdf
27. Clarke, E.M., Grumberg, O., Peled, D.: Model Checking. MIT Press (1999)
28. Leuschel, M., Butler, M.: Prob: A model checker for B. In: Araki, K., Gnesi, S., Mandrioli, D. (eds.) FME 2003. LNCS, vol. 2805, pp. 855–874. Springer, Heidelberg (2003)
29. Macedo, H.D., Larsen, P.G., Fitzgerald, J.: Incremental Development of a Distributed Real-Time Model of a Cardiac Pacing System Using VDM. In: Cuellar, J., Maibaum, T. (eds.) FM 2008. LNCS, vol. 5014, pp. 181–197. Springer, Heidelberg (2008)
30. Gomes, A.O., Oliveira, M.V.M.: Formal specification of a cardiac pacing system. In: Cavalcanti, A., Dams, D.R. (eds.) FM 2009. LNCS, vol. 5850, pp. 692–707. Springer, Heidelberg (2009)
31. Project RODIN: Rigorous open development environment for complex systems (2004), http://rodin-b-sharp.sourceforge.net/

Model-Based Solution for Controlling Physiology

Elthon Oliveira[1,2], Leandro Silva[1,2], Hyggo Almeida[2], and Angelo Perkusich[2]

[1] Universidade Federal de Alagoas
Núcleo de Ciências Exatas - NCEx / Lab. de Computação Pervasiva - Percomp
Campus Arapiraca / Instituto de Computação, Arapiraca / Maceió - Alagoas, Brasil
elthon@arapiraca.ufal.br, leandrodias@ic.ufal.br
[2] Universidade Federal de Campina Grande
Laboratório de Sistemas Embarcados e Computação Pervasiva - Embedded
Centro de Engenharia Elétrica e Informática, Campina Grande - PB, Brasil
hyggo@dsc.ufcg.edu.br, perkusic@dee.ufcg.edu.br

Abstract. In 2008, 63% of the estimated global deaths was due to non-communicable diseases (NCD). One of the main known NCD behavioral risk factors is physical inactivity. Daily physical activity allows controlling weight, reducing NCD death risks. However, irresponsible practice of physical activities can harm both healthy and unhealthy people due to physiological disturbance. In this paper a model-based solution is presented for controlling human physiology during exercise. The presence of non-invasive sensors for collecting physiological data periodically is assumed. Such data is evaluated in comparison to a supervised reference model built using a formal language. Some challenges are also outlined.

Keywords: supervisory control theory, physiology, physical activity.

1 Introduction

According to World Health Organization (WHO) [1], 63% of the estimated global deaths in 2008 were due to non-communicable diseases (NCD). The main known NCD behavioral risk factors are tobacco use, physical inactivity, unhealthy diet and harmful use of alcohol. Daily physical activity allows controlling weight and reduction of cardiovascular disease, type 2 diabetes and cancer risks [2]. Thus, one can say that daily physical activity allows reducing NCD death risks.

Despite the benefits, some risks must be considered while doing regular activity: musculoskeletal injury, dehydration, heat stroke, sudden cardiac death and oxidative stress [3]. Such risks are often experienced with unsupervised and irresponsible practice of physical activities. They can be harmful to both healthy and unhealthy people due to some physiological disturbance. In order to prevent such a disturbance, it is required to strictly follow recommendations from healthcare professionals or to have some professional supervising the exercise.

These life style recommendations are given to patients by healthcare professionals and they are tailored to individual needs based on factors such as age and health status [4]. For instance, suppose a 50 years old patient named Eric with some cardiovascular disease and a 21 years old completely healthy patient named

J. Weber and I. Perseil (Eds.): FHIES 2012, LNCS 7789, pp. 167–175, 2013.

Scott. A heart rate greater than 100 bpm (beats per minute) during a resistance training may represent to Eric a very dangerous situation while to Scott may not. The recommendation to Eric at the right moment his heart rate exceeds 100 bpm could be *"decrease the intensity of the exercise"* or even *"quit exercising"*. Similar recommendations to Scott could be taken at a different threshold.

Once the patient has access to his physiological data during physical activity by means of sensors throughout his body, he would have to keep in mind all the recommendations about the specified limits for all the relevant variables defined for him. Considering just body information, it would already be difficult to reason about. To make it worse, information about the environment, such as temperature or even altitude, may be also relevant depending on the context. As stated in [5] and [6], environmental variables may infect physiology. So, in certain scenarios, different classes of variables (physiological, environmental and behavioral) can be put together in order to take more accurate decisions.

The ideal scenario is that where healthcare professionals personally supervise the patient during his physical activity and keep such a supervision during the recovery period [7]. Despite of being an important procedure, individual supervision is not feasible due to the ratio of *healthcare professionals* to *patients*. Professionals examine patients and give them recommendations of behavior. There is no supervision. Computational solutions for *in loco* physiological monitoring/controlling should mitigate this problem.

In this paper it is presented an approach for controlling human physiology during exercises practice using pervasive computing [8] and supervisory control theory [9]. The presence of non-invasive sensors for collecting physiological (e.g., blood pressure, temperature) and environmental (e.g., altitude, relative humidity) data periodically is assumed. Such data is evaluated in comparison to a supervised reference model built using a formal language. This supervised reference model will represent the knowledge of healthcare professionals (prescription/goal) to control one specific physiological system given the individual profile, his physical activity and the environment where he will be exercising.

Regular automata are the chosen formal language used with supervisory control due to its simplicity and expressiveness. Besides, each part of the system (variables) can be modeled separately. Then, a bigger and more complex model representing the whole system can be obtained from the product operation executed over the smaller models. Such an operation is automatically performed. In this way, in the case of change in one the variables, just a specific small model must be manually changed. A new system model can be generated again by applying the mentioned operation. In comparison to a common rule-based style system, it is easier to promote changes into the reference model.

2   Defining the Human Physiology Control

Physiological state can be seen as a set of values of all physiological variables that can assume any value within their respective defined ranges. For instance, assuming intervals for heart rate $[70, 100)$ (meaning *good_h*) and $[100, +\infty)$ (meaning *bad_h*), and for systolic blood pressure [90, 119] (meaning *good_p*) and (119, +∞) (meaning *bad_p*). An individual with a 110 bpm heart rate and a 95 mmHg systolic blood pressure would present {*bad_h,good_p*} as his physiological state.

The state of individual may not only be composed by physiological variables, but it can also be enriched with the other two classes of variables: environmental and behavioral ones. Besides, events like *slow down* or *breath slowly* could change the state of the individual from {*bad_h,good_p*} to {*good_h,good_p*}. Some of these events are known by healthcare professionals and are passed to patients as recommendations like *"if you are running and your heart rate is greater than 100 bpm, slow down a bit"*. Three parts are observed in this recommendation: (i) a behavioral information (*running*), (ii) a physiological information (*heart rate is greater than 100 bpm*) and (iii) an event (*slow down a bit*). The event (or action) *slow down a bit* can be controlled and should be taken by the patient so its heart rate can also be controlled, consequently. In Figure 1, a finite state machine (FSM) that represents this scenario is presented. The arrow pointing to state *good_h.good_p* indicates that it is the initial state of the "machine".

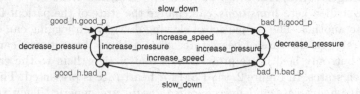

Fig. 1. FSM with two variables

Based on this recommendation format, the set of states and the events can be seen as a discrete event system (DES) [10]. And like all DES, it can be controlled at some operation levels.

2.1 Steps for Defining the Control

Defining human physiological control consists of five steps. Each step must be followed based on the previous ones. Such steps must be executed by a healthcare professional during anamnesis. The steps are detailed bellow.

1. **Delineating the Individual Profile.** The healthcare professional must:
   - identify if the patient is affected by some disease (chronic or not);
   - measure all important variables (heart rate, blood sugar, etc);
   - define the patient goal (prevention, treatment, training, etc);
   - classify the patient according to his physical condition (sedentary, common athlete, high performance athlete, etc); and
   - identify the environments where the patient can do his physical activities (outdoor, indoor, ate a gym, at home, etc).

2. **Defining Variables to Monitor and/or Control.**
Not all variables must be monitored in every case. Some variables may be important and some others may be considered irrelevant depending on the patient profile, the environment and the expected behavior. For instance, in a resistive training, *speed* is irrelevant. The three classes of variables that can be monitored and/or controlled are:

   - physiological: heart rate, body temperature, blood sugar, etc;
   - environmental: temperature, relative humidity, altitude, etc; and
   - behavioral: standing, sitting, lying, running, walking, etc.

3. **Defining Intervals of Values for Each Chosen Variable.**
It is necessary to define the intervals of values for each chosen variable and name them. Any interval can be defined and this should be done based on each case. For instance, assume the need of a FSM with only two states. Following the rules described by CDC[1], the heart rate intervals to **moderate-intensity** and **vigorous-intensity** physical activities of a 50 years old patient should be in $[85, 119]$ and $[120, 144]$, respectively. The number of states and what rules to follow depend on the needs and specificities of each case.

4. **Defining Events/Actions between the Defined States.**
Events, called here *transitions*, can change the state of the patient from one state to another. The simple act of slowing down when jogging can decrease heart rate. In the case of heart rate, more actions (transitions) can do the same, but only healthcare professionals may assign them to the transition between states. In Figure 2, the FSM for heart rate is presented. The events *increase_heart_rate* and *decrease_heart_rate* are generic. They represent actions/recommendations that change state of patient heart rate.

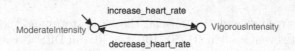

Fig. 2. FSM for heart hate

5. **Defining the Specification According to the Patient Goal.**
People that seek for a healthcare professional have different goals. They may look for physical activity as prescription for some disease treatment, for disease prevention, or for a healthy way of physical improvement. In all these cases, patients must follow recommendations given by the healthcare professional. In this approach, recommendations are described as automata and/or some automata concepts like *forbidden state* and *accepting state*. An example will be illustrated in Section 2.3.

It is important to highlight that all these steps must be followed by a healthcare professional. Even with some clinical guidelines in hand, one must have the

---

[1] Centers of Disease Control and Prevention (http://www.cdc.gov).

domain knowledge and experience with real cases so the model can express, at the worst case, almost all of (and only) the relevant features of the case.

2.2   User/Model Interaction

As stated before, the presence of non-invasive sensors is assumed. Each one of the three classes of variable may be monitored by a specific sensor that collects their data periodically. The reading periodicity depends on the nature of the variable. So, one variable may be read in every five seconds and another may be read in every 20 minutes. Collected data are sent to a server to be processed.

Desktop PCs, tablets or even smartphones can be used as servers. After processing data, server must send feedback to patient. Any kind of device with a display (e.g.; cellphone, TV, treadmill) can receive data and be used to show feedback messages to patient. In the case of server being a smartphone, messages may be showed by itself without the need to send data to another entity.

Every time a variable is read, a two columns table (with variables and their last collected values) is updated. The current state of the system, represented by the value-column, is located in one state of the reference model. If such a state is considered desirable, an "ok" message is given to patient. Otherwise, a "not ok" message with a sequence of actions, named path, is given to patient as text messages. It is this path that can take patient from an undesirable state (unsafe or not) to a desirable one. The actions that form path are the labels of transitions that take patient from origin state to destination one.

2.3   An Example

Due to space restrictions, instead of presenting a bigger and more complex case study, it is presented a functional toy example. However, it was intended to show as many details as possible about the approach presented in this work.

In this example it is presented a case where the patient aims to lose weight. For this, he intends to practice jogging regularly.

1. **Delineating the individual profile.**
   A 25-years-old male person with sedentary routine and no history of disease.
2. **Defining variables to monitor and/or control.**
   It is planned to monitor and control *hear rate* and *systolic blood pressure* variables. Environmental and behavioral variables are not considered here.
3. **Defining intervals of values for each chosen variable.**
   Due to didactic purposes, the number of states for each chosen variable is small. States and their intervals are presented in Table 1.
4. **Defining events/actions between the defined states.**
   Two generic events are defined for each FSM (a.k.a. model). For heart rate model there are *increase_heart_rate* and *decrease_heart_rate* (Figure 3(a)). And for systolic blood pressure model there are *increase_pressure* and *decrease_pressure* (Figure 3(b)). As aforesaid, each one of the generic events

Table 1. States and their intervals of the chosen variables

Variable	State	Interval
Heart rate (bpm)	safe	$[97, 156]$
	tolerable	$[157, 175]$
	dangerous	$[176, 195]$
Systolic blood pressure (mmHg)	hypotension	$[-\infty, 89]$
	desirable	$[90, 119]$
	prehypertension	$[120, 139]$
	hypertension	$[140, +\infty]$

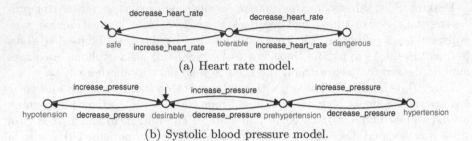

(a) Heart rate model.

(b) Systolic blood pressure model.

Fig. 3. FSM's for the chosen variables

can be replaced by a set of actions/recommendations. For instance, depending on the context, *increase_pressure* could be replaced by events such as *increase_environmental_temperature*, *increase_speed* or *eat_salty_food*.

5. **Defining the specification according to the patient goal.**
   The recommendations that patient must follow are: (i) the blood pressure cannot decrease from its initial state and (ii) if the blood pressure increases, it must decrease. It is aimed to keep the patient in a set of physiological states in where he can be safe during his physical activity.

   Specifications can be written by two ways. One is building an automaton that works as a constraint (Figure 4). Another way is by setting some states as *forbidden*, but it is not presented here due to space restrictions.

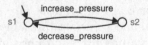

Fig. 4. Specification for systolic blood pressure

At first, after executing all five steps, it is enough to make a product of the models defined after the 4th step. The outcome model possess states that represent all the combinations among states from the two models. The outcome model has 12 states and 34 transitions.

Then, applying the product to this outcome model and the specification, a supervised model is produced. This new model contains only 6 states and 14 transitions that follow the written specifications/recommendations (Figure 5). The states are painted gray indicating that all of them are *accepting states*.

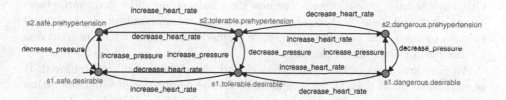

Fig. 5. Reference model for patient physiological behavior

The model allows the patient to enter in one of the two *dangerous* physiology states (heart rate between 185 and 195 bpm). If it is desired to avoid such states, in the 5th step it is enough to set the *dangerous* state, from the *hear rate* model, as a *forbidden* state.

3   Related Work

Many works have been developed in the area of pervasive healthcare in the last years. Almost all of them concern about disease diagnosis and others about disease and medication treatments [11].

Some works focus on diagnostic algorithms. Most of them are about cardiac diseases. The ones that stand out are developed for atrial fibrillation [12], myocardial infarction and atrio-ventricular block [13] and cardiac arrhythmia [14]. Others focus on different kinds of diseases. The work presented by [15] uses neural networks for diagnosing diabetes. The one presented by [16] proposes the development of a diagnoses system of sleep apnea and hypopnea syndrome. And in [17], a pervasive and preventive healthcare solution addressing the medication noncompliance is proposed.

None of these works focus on disease prevention and treatment with data fusion (different classes of variables). There is a proposal of a fusion data model [18], but it does not include behavioral and environmental information. One work deals with different classes of variables [19]. However, due to the decision rules format, there is no efficient support for evolution of the model.

There is a commercial tool (http://www.bodymedia.com/) in the context of exercises practice. However, its purpose is to count calories consumed during activities executed by user daily and supervise him to lose weight.

4   Final Remarks

In this work an approach to promote safe and controlled physical activities based on models is presented. A deeper research into the supervisory control theory is intended to be done to promote a more accurate control of human physiology. In this way, unanticipated human behavior and some real world constraints omitted here can be overcome in more complex and real scenarios.

This work focuses on control of human physiology. It can be used to monitoring exercise aiming disease prevention or treatment, and physical improvement. Other potential applications are medication management, diet program, emergency alert and identification of conflicts among recommendations. As formal models are used, it is possible to generate verified source code which is great due to the level of demanded reliability.

An easy evolution of the human model and also data fusion are promoted. It is enough to build a FSM for a new variable and apply the product operation with the rest of the models. Besides, each model can be completely customized. One can say that the models are individual-physiology-profile oriented.

An new step or phase is added to clinical workflow. A healthcare supervisor *controls* and/or *gives suggestions to* patient all the time to prevent his physiological system to not follow recommendations given by human professional.

The periodicity in which sensors read variables must be set by the heath care professional. Each variable should be read in a different period due to its specific characteristics. The accuracy of controlling must increase with short periods.

The non-friendly interface of automata is a problem. Another drawback is the necessary formal minimum knowledge. As this work is still conceptual, such disadvantages are not critical since friendly software interfaces are intended.

It is clear that building such a reference model will represent an additional time in clinical workflow execution. In this way, efforts must be employed to develop tools that mitigate necessary time for this task. Besides, as it was mentioned in Section 2.3, the generated reference model presents all the possible combinations of states. Medical knowledge (in some structured way) will be used to prune models so that no physiologically impossible states remain.

Validation of this work will be conducting together with the healthcare professional. At first, this will be done with simulated data. A program to be developed will interact with reference model supplying physiological, environmental and behavioral information. Messages exchanged between them will be analysed by the human professional. Later, generated source-code will be embedded in some devices and the work will be submitted to real test on the field. Nevertheless, it will be necessary to acquire sensors with some communication features. With this, it is intended to demonstrate the feasibility of this work concept. It is also intended to define a more realistic example so it can be used as a full case study. This more realistic example will demand the presence of a healthcare professional for following the described steps to build the formal reference model.

References

1. World Health Organization: World health statistics. WHO Press (2012)
2. Bianchini, F., Kaaks, R., Vainio, H.: Weight control and physical activity in cancer prevention. Obesity Reviews 3(1), 5–8 (2002)

3. Melzer, K., Kayser, B., Pichard, C.: Physical activity: the health benefits outweigh the risks. Current Opinion in Clinical Nutrition and Metabolic Care 7(6), 641–647 (2004) PMID: 15534432
4. Fletcher, G., Trejo, J.F.: Why and how to prescribe exercise: Overcoming the barriers. Cleveland Clinic Journal of Medicine 72(8), 645–649 (2005)
5. Wilmshurst, P.: Temperature and cardiovascular mortality. BMJ 309(6961), 1029–1030 (1994)
6. Fujiwara, T., Kawamura, M., Nakajima, J., Adachi, T., Hiramori, K.: Seasonal differences in diurnal blood pressure of hypertensive patients living in a stable environmental temperature. Journal of Hypertension 13(12), 1747–1752 (1995)
7. American College of Sports and Medicine: ACSM's Guidelines for Exercise Testing and Prescription, 6th edn. Lippincott Williams & Wilkins (February 2000)
8. Weiser, M.: The computer for the 21st century. Scientific American (February 1991)
9. Ramadge, P.J., Wonham, W.M.: The control of discrete event systems. Proceedings of the IEEE 77(1), 81–98 (1989)
10. Cassandras, C.G., Lafortune, S.: Introduction to Discrete Event Systems, 1 edn. Springer (September 1999)
11. Koutkias, V.G., Chouvarda, I., Triantafyllidis, A., Malousi, A., Giaglis, G.D., Maglaveras, N.: A personalized framework for medication treatment management in chronic care. IEEE Transactions on Information Technology in Biomedicine: A Publication of the IEEE Engineering in Medicine and Biology Society 14(2), 464–472 (2010) PMID: 20007042
12. Yaghouby, F., Ayatollahi, A., Bahramali, R., Yaghouby, M., Alavi, A.H.: Towards automatic detection of atrial fibrillation: A hybrid computational approach. Computers in Biology and Medicine 40(11-12), 919–930 (2010)
13. Sankari, Z., Adeli, H.: HeartSaver: a mobile cardiac monitoring system for auto-detection of atrial fibrillation, myocardial infarction, and atrio-ventricular block. Computers in Biology and Medicine 41(4), 211–220 (2011) PMID: 21377149
14. Özçift, A.: Random forests ensemble classifier trained with data resampling strategy to improve cardiac arrhythmia diagnosis. Computers in Biology and Medicine 41(5), 265–271 (2011)
15. Karan, O., Bayraktar, C., Gümüşkaya, H., Karlık, B.: Diagnosing diabetes using neural networks on small mobile devices. Expert Syst. Appl. 39(1), 54–60 (2012)
16. Burgos, A., Goñi, A., Illarramendi, A., Bermudez, J.: Real-Time detection of apneas on a PDA. IEEE Transactions on Information Technology in Biomedicine 14(4), 995–1002 (2010)
17. Pang, Z., Chen, Q., Zheng, L.: A pervasive and preventive healthcare solution for medication noncompliance and daily monitoring. In: 2nd International Symp. on Appl. Sciences in Biomedical and Communication Technologies, pp. 1–6 (November 2009)
18. Pantelopoulos, A., Bourbakis, N.G.: Prognosis-a wearable health-monitoring system for people at risk: methodology and modeling. IEEE Transactions on Information Technology in Biomedicine: A Publication of the IEEE Engineering in Medicine and Biology Society 14(3), 613–621 (2010) PMID: 20123575
19. Copetti, A., Leite, J.C.B., Loques, O.: A decision mechanism to context inference in pervasive healthcare environments. SBA: Controle e Automação Sociedade Brasileira de Automática 22(4), 363–378 (2011)

Automated Reviewing of Healthcare Security Policies

Nafees Qamar[1], Johannes Faber[1], Yves Ledru[2], and Zhiming Liu[1]

[1] United Nations University
International Institute for Software Technology
{nqamar,jfaber,lzm}@iist.unu.edu
[2] UJF-Grenoble 1/Grenoble-INP/UPMF-Grenoble2/CNRS, LIG
yves.ledru@imag.fr

Abstract. We present a new formal validation method for healthcare security policies in the form of feedback-based queries to ensure an answer to the question of *Who* is accessing *What* in Electronic Health Records. To this end, we consider Role-based Access Control (RBAC) that offers the flexibility to specify the users, roles, permissions, actions, and the objects to secure. We use the Z notation both for formal specification of RBAC security policies and for queries aimed at reviewing these security policies. To ease the effort in creating the correct specification of the security policies, RBAC-based graphical models (such as SecureUML) are used and automatically translated into the corresponding Z specifications. These specifications are then animated using the Jaza tool to execute queries against the specification of security policies. Through this process, it is automatically detected who will gain access to the medical record of the patient and which information will be exposed to that system user.

1 Introduction

Security and privacy in information systems generally concern questions such as *Who accesses What.* An Electronic Health Record (EHR) is a longitudinal electronic record of health information for a patient generated by one or more encounters in any care delivery setting. Security mechanisms are supposed to be applied to protect such EHRs to shield against *external threats* from outside the system, such as attacking or running malicious applications, as well as *internal threats* from inside the system, e.g., a valid system user illegitimately accesses private data of a patient. It was, however, reported that major threats to patient privacy actually stemmed mostly from internal factors [Jou09]. For this reason, it is essential to investigate who is doing what in a system besides ensuring smooth data availability. For example, what are the operations a user such as a nurse can perform, and what resources are accessible by a user? The system also needs to be flexible enough to allow exceptional access to system resources, especially in medical emergency cases. Due to these exceptions, the large number of stakeholders, end users, and interaction components, the specification of policies

J. Weber and I. Perseil (Eds.): FHIES 2012, LNCS 7789, pp. 176–193, 2013.
© Springer-Verlag Berlin Heidelberg 2013

on security and privacy and their correct implementation in EHR systems are particularly challenging. Not surprisingly, medical data disclosure is the second highest reported breach [HY06]. To address this issue, legal regulations, such as USA's Health Care Insurance Portability and Accountability Act (HIPAA), are in place as safeguards to confidentiality, integrity, and availability of these systems.

To guarantee that application-specific security objectives are enforced by the enacted security policies based on regulations like HIPAA, the rules that define the security policies need to be justified using validation techniques. To this end, we propose using the Z notation [Spi92, DW96] to represent the security rules as well as to specify queries for revealing internal threats to EHRs. The execution of the queries animates the security policies to generate feedbacks on authorized and unauthorized states of an EHR system. Additionally, these also help in analyzing over- or under-designed security policies, which otherwise can block desirable operations or permit undesirable ones, respectively.

To ease the effort in model construction and understanding, we propose to use a graphical notation, such as SecureUML [LBD02] or UMLsec [Jür05], to model security policies. The graphical models are automatically translated into specifications in the formal Z notation, which is amenable to formal analysis. In this way, the proposed formal approach can be integrated with graphical modeling and transformation techniques – the so-called model-driven techniques. For specifying security policies, we apply the standardized Role-based Access Control (RBAC) mechanism [FSG+01]. RBAC offers roles, which are permanent organizational positions whilst users can arbitrarily be changed. Based on this, we introduce formalized review functions in terms of Z specifications. These review functions can be animated using, e.g., the Jaza tool to get feedback on which actions are available to which role, on access to specific resources, and on duplicate permissions. To further reflect the complex situation in the healthcare domain, we additionally introduce Separation of Duties (SoD) constraints to analyze conflicts of interest between different stakeholders in the system. This is done statically, by ensuring that a user cannot have two conflicting roles at all, as well as dynamically, by ensuring that a user cannot have two conflicting roles in a single session. We exemplary demonstrate that this approach is suitable to deal with emergency situations, where immediate access to information might be needed and report on the types of information one needs to collect before deploying a security policy. We prefer RBAC to Mandatory Access Control [BL75] and Discretionary Access Control [DOD85], because it builds on a generic principle of access control that makes it adaptable to any organizational structure and flexible with respect to the application implementation.

To summarize, we present a new formal validation method for healthcare security policies with two main contributions. First, we introduce formally specified queries for automatically reviewing security policies and analyze what information of an EHR is exposed to a system user. Second, we introduce SoD constraints to cope with the complex security policies usually found in EHR systems. We use an example from the healthcare domain for demonstration.

The paper is structured as follows: Section 2 discusses state-of-the-art formal techniques on security policies. Section 3 states RBAC and gives a scenario, which is used as a running example throughout the paper. Section 4 demonstrates the formalization of security policies in Z notation, whereas Sect. 5 presents formally specified queries for reviewing security policies. Section 6 formalizes SoD constraints, and finally, Sect. 7 concludes and shares some perspectives.

2   Related Work

Healthcare privacy and security techniques are intended to cope with a number of issues such as authorized data disclosure, integrity of information, regulatory implication for healthcare, and information security risk management. The survey [AJ10] also considers a multitude of such techniques and provides a classification. The authors conclude that existing techniques are inadequate to meet security and privacy challenges in EHRs. It also shows that healthcare security and privacy issues have not been treated in a deserved manner. Our findings complement this survey concerning these issues, which also have not been dealt with formal languages such as the Z notation, generally known for their precision and unambiguity. For example, [TMB06] uses formal methods to improve medical protocols, but such techniques are missing in general.

The standardized Z notation [Spi92] has been successfully applied to various industrial projects for formal modeling and development [Bow03]. Our past work presents an RBAC-based security kernel using Z [QLI11, LQI+11], which shows that Z can be effectively used to verify or validate security policies. The work in this paper builds on these preliminary results with an extended set of formal queries for validation of security policies and formal SoD constraints. The use of Z in our previous work is motivated by the support of authorization constraints, which do not appear in this paper. When there are authorization constraints, one needs to consider the evolution of the state of the functional model [LIM+11]. Currently, only our tool takes this evolution in the animation of the complete model into account.

Alloy has the potential to do similar work as Z, but currently no tool is available covering both functional security models and authorization constraints. Regarding B, a similar tool is currently under development in the Selkis project [MIL+11]. The tool will allow using the ProB tool both for animation and model checking.

ISO-standardized RBAC has widely been described by researchers using Z such as [Hal94, AK06, YHHZ06]. However, the work there offers only generic formal representation of RBAC. There are other techniques for validation and verification of security properties [MSGC07, Bos95, AK06]. In particular, [MSGC07] proposes a process to verify Z specifications by the Z/EVES theorem prover. In parallel, OCL expressions are also meant to specify restrictions on a system model but do not support feedback queries. For example, SecureMOVA [BCDE09] offers a set of queries to analyze security policies expressed as formulas in UML's Object Constraint Language.

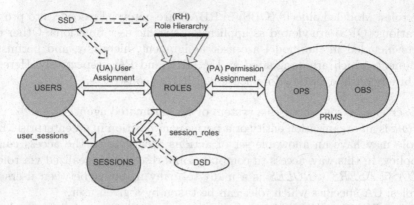

Fig. 1. Role Based Access Control [FSG+01]

The work [ZWCJ02] proposes to verify algebraic characteristics of RBAC schemas using Alloy. Alloy is used as a constraint analyzer to check the inconsistencies among roles and Static Separation of Duty (SSD) constraints and to generate a counter-example when inconsistencies are found. However, the work addresses SSD constraints only. [SM02, AH07] also discuss SoD constraints. The former discusses decentralized administration of RBAC and allows arbitrary changes to an initially stated model that may result in conflicting policies over time with respect to SoD constraints. They argue that SoD constraints may introduce implicit security policy flaws because of role hierarchies. In [TRA+09], a translation from UML to Alloy is given for verification of the UML models. The work is mainly focused on analysis of contextual information such as location and time for access decisions.

3   Role-Based Access Control

In this section, we introduce the preliminaries of Role-based Access Control (RBAC). We will use a running example to illustrate the basic concepts and properties.

3.1   Data Model of RBAC

The data model of RBAC [FSG+01] as shown in Fig. 1 is based on five data types: users (USERS), roles (ROLES), objects (OBS), permissions (PRMS) and executable operations (OPS) by users on objects. A sixth data type for sessions (SESSIONS) is used to associate roles temporarily to users. Sessions correspond to the dynamic aspect of RBAC that actually includes session management.

RBAC differentiates between users and roles. A role is considered as a permanent position in an organization whereas a given user might be switched with another user for that role. Thus, *rights* are offered to roles instead of users. Roles are assigned to permissions that can later be exercised by users playing these roles. Modeled objects (OBS) in RBAC are potential resources to protect. Operations (OPS) are viewed as application-specific user functions. Other constructs included in the model are user assignment, hierarchy, and permission assignment, which are designated as UA, RH, and PA, respectively. Here, we very briefly outline all the aforementioned RBAC constructs:

- *User* is a person who uses a system or an automated agent.
- *Role* is an organization entity or a permanent position in an enterprise. Each role may have an allowable set of actions according to the access control policy. In this way, access to computational resources is realized via roles.
- $UA \subseteq USERS \times ROLES$ is a many-to-many mapping between users and roles; UA specifies which roles can be taken by a given user.
- $PA \subseteq PRMS \times ROLES$ is a many-to-many mapping permission-to-role; PA expresses which roles may be granted a given permission.
- $user\_sessions(u : USERS) \rightarrow 2^{SESSIONS}$ is a mapping of user u onto a set of sessions; it lists the current sessions of a given user.
- $session\_roles(s : SESSIONS) \rightarrow 2^{ROLES}$ is a mapping of session s onto a set of roles; it lists the current roles of a given user in a given session.
- $RH \subseteq ROLES \times ROLES$ is a partially ordered role hierarchy; a senior role may inherit the permissions from its junior roles.
- $PRMS : 2^{OPS \times OBS}$ is a set of permissions. Permissions are regarded as an approval to perform operations on RBAC-protected objects. An executable image of a program is considered as an operation, which executes some function for the user. For example, within medical records, operations might include insert, delete, append, and update medical instructions.

3.2   Example: RBAC-Based Security Management for EHRs

Healthcare security policies are ideally modeled using RBAC, because permanent positions such as doctors, nurses, and other healthcare staff can be mapped to the roles as set in the policy. Figure 2 represents a small healthcare security policy management, which attempts to secure medical records by the use of roles associated to permissions given as stereotypes, while permissions are on the class i.e., MedicalRecords. For instance, a patient, which corresponds to a particular role in an EHR system, has the ability to read his/her own medical record. A doctor inherits permissions from the patient, besides holding another permission given as UserCredentials, on which the doctor could exercise a write operation. The role EmergencyOfficer is assigned with a permission such as read, which is intended for emergency access. Using our toolset [LQI+11] one can translate such diagram into a Z model. Here we confine ourselves to explain the needed part to allow reviewing of such formal translations.

Access Control Violations. Access control rules specified as graphical models are hard to validate because of their ambiguous semantics. This in turn leads to information integrity and confidentiality problems in general. In the example

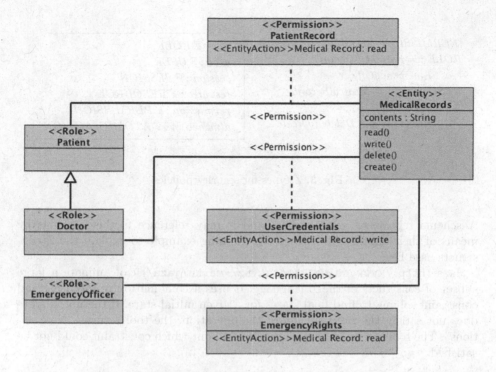

Fig. 2. Design of a medical application using SecureUML

above, a patient could change his/her own medical record if the security policy is not correctly realized in the system. Similarly, a doctor being also a patient can forge his/her own medical record if not avoided by a corresponding SoD constraint. To address these inadequate security policies, we introduce a technique for automatically reviewing such deficiencies in Sect. 5 after the next section's discussion on the formalization of policies.

4   Formalized Healthcare Security Policies

This section gives an overview of the formalization of security policies, which has been introduced in our previous work [QLI11].

4.1   The Z Notation and the Jaza Tool

The ISO-standardized Z language [Spi92] offers an extensive set of concepts and constructs from first-order logic and set theory to specify software systems. Schemas are the major structuring primitives in Z. Each schema is further divided into two components: the signature part, which includes variables and types, and the predicate part, for imposing constraints upon these variables.

$$[PERMISSION, SESSION, USER]$$
$$ROLE ::= Patient \mid Doctor \mid$$
$$\quad EmergencyOfficer$$
$$RESOURCE ::= MedicalRecords$$
$$ATOMIC\_ACTION ::=$$
$$\quad Read \mid Write \mid Delete \mid Create$$

___ Sets _____
$role : \mathbb{F}\ ROLE$
$user : \mathbb{F}\ USER$
$session : \mathbb{F}\ SESSION$
$resource : \mathbb{F}\ RESOURCE$
$permission : \mathbb{F}\ PERMISSION$
$atm\_action : \mathbb{F}\ ATOMIC\_ACTION$

Fig. 3. Z types for security policies

A schema represents an operation, and it may reference further schemas by means of their names. We will use the running example to explain the Z constructs used here.

Jaza (http://www.cs.waikato.ac.nz/~marku/jaza/) can animate a large subset of constructs of the Z language. It uses a combination of rewriting and constraint solving to find final states for a given initial state. If the initial state does not satisfy the precondition of the operation, the tool returns "No Solutions". The tool can be further queried to find out which constraint could not be satisfied.

4.2 Z Models for Security Policies

We explain our formalization of security policies with the Z notation following the example from Sect. 3.2. This approach from [QLI11] can be used to formalize security policies following the RBAC data model as given in Sect. 3.1.

Z Schemas. Using Z, six types are introduced in Fig. 3 as basic type definitions (PERMISSION, SESSION, USER) or enumerated types on the left. The value of these types is based on the security model presented in Fig. 2. The schema Sets on the right side declares corresponding finite sets ($\mathbb{F}$) for each of these types.

Jaza Representation. The following Jaza expressions initialize some of these sets according to the values of the running example from Sect. 3.2.

```
atm_action' == {Read, Write, Delete, Create},
permission' == {"PatientRecord", "UserCredentials", "EmergencyRights"},
resource' == {MedicalRecords},
role' == {Patient, Doctor, EmergencyOfficer},
user' == {"Alice", "Bob", "Mark"},
```

The schema Perm_Assignment reminds of the underlying translation from graphical SecureUML models to Z notation. It is used to compute the table perm_Assignment in Fig. 4. In [QLI11] this schema as well as the translation of SecureUML models in general are explained. One can also find there the corresponding rules to automatically generate other RBAC structures such as PA, UA, sessions, and role hierarchy. For this work, it is sufficient to understand the type of the resulting permission assignment as shown in the following schema: users with assigned roles are related to a set of permissions for specific resources.

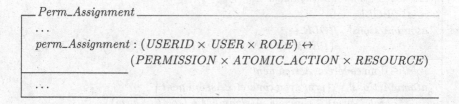

The table perm_Assignment, pictured in Fig. 4 in Jaza syntax, results from the translation process. It creates a link between a user's ID, users and their assigned roles to the permissions, the operations, and the resources. The set for user IDs (USERID) is not available in RBAC, but we believe it will be useful when implementing a real system. This generated table assigns the initial permission values for the use with a Z-based formal model animator such as Jaza.

This sums up the formalization of the access control information for the running example, which can be interpreted by a tool. In the following, we present formal queries allowing us to analyze suchlike formal models for security rules.

5 Formal Queries for Healthcare Security Policies

The RBAC model provides mainly three types of functions to operate on security policies: administrative, supporting system, and review. *Administrative functions* involve creation and maintenance of basic sets of elements. These sets are USERS, ROLES, OPS and OBS. Additionally, constructing relations among the sets is also supported by administrative functions (UA and PA assignments). This has already been covered in an earlier paper [QLI11].

Review Functions, on the other hand, help in querying the data structures such as those of UA and PA assignments. The administrator may view the contents of specified relations through review functions. By this means, we can perform queries to request the users assigned to a role, permissions of a role, and allowed roles in a session. In the RBAC standard, the review functions are either mandatory, like querying the assigned users and assigned roles, or optional, like querying permissions of a role. Therefore, not all RBAC implementations provide all review functions. In the following, we present a set of formalized and extended review functions, which provide feedback on the contents of the security policies.

5.1 Authorized Roles for an Atomic Action

The first operation schema EvaluateRoleAuthorizedAtomicAction computes the
set of atomic actions for a given role. This query is helpful when one needs to
evaluate who can perform a particular operation in a given security policy.

$$
\begin{array}{l}
\rule{3cm}{0.4pt}\ EvaluateRoleAuthorizedAtomicAction \rule{4cm}{0.4pt} \\
\Xi\,Sets\,;\ \Xi\,ComputeAssignment \\
role? : ROLE \\
atomicActions! : ROLE \leftrightarrow \\
\qquad\qquad (PERMISSION \times ATOMIC\_ACTION \times RESOURCE) \\
\rule{6cm}{0.4pt} \\
role? \in \mathrm{dom}\ concrete\_Assignment \\
atomicActions! = \{prm : \mathrm{ran}\ concrete\_Assignment\ | \\
\qquad (role?, prm) \in concrete\_Assignment \bullet (role? \mapsto prm)\}
\end{array}
$$

The declaration part of a Z schema is notated above the horizontal line,
whereas the predicate part below the horizontal line defines constraints on the declared variables. The declaration part of the schema EvaluateRoleAuthorizedAtomicAction includes the state schema Sets (the symbol Ξ basically indicates that
its elements are not changed in this schema) and an input variable role? of type
ROLE. The output set being computed, atomicActions! (i.e., operations from a
modeled system), is a relation that is a cross product of a role with associated
permissions, atomic actions, and resources. The predicate part of the schema
checks that the input role (role?) is actually from the domain of the relation
concrete_Assignment. The output (atomicActions!) is the set of all possible values
associated with a particular role (i.e., role?). Note that concrete_Assignment is
actually defined in a further schema ComputeAssignment, which is not shown
here in full detail due to space reasons, but can be found in [QLI11].

$$
\begin{array}{l}
\rule{3cm}{0.4pt}\ ComputeAssignment \rule{5cm}{0.4pt} \\
\ldots \\
concrete\_Assignment : ROLE \leftrightarrow \\
\qquad\qquad (PERMISSION \times ATOMIC\_ACTION \times RESOURCE) \\
\rule{6cm}{0.4pt} \\
\ldots
\end{array}
$$

The set construction in schema EvaluateRoleAuthorizedAtomicAction

$$
\{prm : \mathrm{ran}\ concrete\_Assignment\ | \\
\qquad (role?, prm) \in concrete\_Assignment \bullet (role? \mapsto prm)\}
$$

first declares a local variable prm to be in the range of concrete_Assignment. The
predicate part, $(role?, prm) \in concrete\_Assignment$, selects tuples of the shape
$(role?, prm)$ occurring in concrete_Assignment. Finally, the expression behind

```
perm_Assignment ==
{
  (("ABC001", "Alice", Patient, ("PatientRecord", Read, MedicalRecords)),
  (("ABC002", "Bob", Doctor, ("PatientRecord", Read, MedicalRecords)),
  (("ABC003", "Bob", Doctor, ("UserCredentials", Write, MedicalRecords)),
  (("ABC004", " Mark", EmergencyOfficer,
                            ("EmergencyRights", Read, MedicalRecords)),
},
```

Fig. 4. Permission assignment in Jaza syntax

the • symbol collects the maplets for all of these permissions in the set. By this
the result relation is built. Below we show an example of executing this schema
against an input role EmergencyOfficer from the running example (cf. Fig. 4).
Jaza lists the operations that the emergency officer is permitted to perform.

```
JAZA> ;EvaluateRoleAuthorizedAtomicAction
  Input role? = EmergencyOfficer
  atomicActions!==
  {(EmergencyOfficer, ("EmergencyRights", Read, MedicalRecords))}
```

5.2   Actions Available for a Role

The operation schema EvaluateActionsAgainstRoles works exactly opposite to the
operation schema EvaluateRoleAuthorizedAtomicAction, which, for a given atomic
action, returns the list of all associated roles (along with a resource and a permission) to perform that action.

_____
$\_EvaluateActionsAgainstRoles\_$
$\Xi Sets$; $\Xi ComputeAssignment$
$atm\_action? : ATOMIC\_ACTION$
$roleAction! : ROLE \leftrightarrow$
$\qquad (PERMISSION \times ATOMIC\_ACTION \times RESOURCE)$
_____
$roleAction! = \{r : \text{dom } comp\_Assignment; \ p : permission; \ rsrc : resource \ |$
$\qquad (r \mapsto (p, atm\_action?, rsrc)) \in concrete\_Assignment \bullet$
$\qquad (r \mapsto (p, atm\_action?, rsrc))\}$
_____

The input (atm_action?) is of the set type ATOMIC_ACTION. The output role-
Action! has the same type as given in the previous schema. The set roleAction!
retrieves the allowed roles to perform an atomic action. Note that we also retrieve the associated permissions and resources with each obtained role since
this appears more comprehensible from a security engineer's point of view. In
the following example of this schema query, we provide an atomic action named
Read, and the corresponding information is returned.

```
JAZA> ;EvaluateActionsAgainstRoles
  Input atm\_action? = Read
  atomicActions!=={(Patient, ("PatientRecord", Read, MedicalRecords)),
  (Doctor, ("PatientRecord", Read, MedicalRecords)), (EmergencyOfficer,
  ("EmergencyRights", Read, MedicalRecords))}
```

5.3   Analyzing Access to a Resource

It is equally important to know the resources within the system that can be accessed by some roles. EvaluateResourcesAccess is used to this end. For a given resource resource?, it returns the pairs of atomic actions associated with that particular resource.

$$
\begin{array}{l}
\underline{EvaluateResourcesAccess} \\[4pt]
\Xi\,Sets;\ \Xi\,ComputeAssignment \\
resource? : RESOURCE \\
resourcesAccess! : ROLE \leftrightarrow \\
\qquad\qquad (PERMISSION \times (ATOMIC\_ACTION \times RESOURCE)) \\
action\_resource\_set! : \mathbb{F}(ATOMIC\_ACTION \times RESOURCE) \\[6pt]
\hline \\
resourcesAccess! = \{r : \mathrm{dom}\ comp\_Assignment;\ p : permission; \\
\qquad\quad atm : atm\_action \mid (r \mapsto (p, atm, resource?)) \\
\qquad\qquad\quad \in concrete\_Assignment \bullet (r \mapsto (p, (atm, resource?)))\} \\
action\_resource\_set! = \{x : \mathrm{ran}\ resourcesAccess! \bullet second(x)\}
\end{array}
$$

This operation also takes an input resource? of the type RESOURCE and computes the related roles and atomic actions of that resource; action_resource_set! ensures that only the atomic actions corresponding to the resources are retrieved. This schema is exemplified below: the input is resource MedicalRecords, and the result produced by Jaza is printed[1].

```
JAZA> ;EvaluateResourcesAccess
  Input resource? = MedicalRecords
  action\_resource\_set!=={(Read, MedicalRecords),(Write,
  MedicalRecords), (Delete, MedicalRecords),(Create, MedicalRecords)}
```

5.4   Permissions for Atomic Action and Role

The operation schema FindPermissions is intended to query the permissions for both a given atomic action and a role. This schema has two input parameters i.e., atm_action? and role? of the types ATOMIC_ACTION and ROLE, respectively. The predicate computes the set of permissions for the input role and the atomic action. As a result, perms! will return the set of all associated permissions for the input values. We need to give the atomic action along with the role as input, and it will return the permissions linked to them.

---

[1] Here and in the following we only show the relevant outputs.

```
┌─ FindPermissions ────────────────────────────────────────
│ ΞSets ; Ξ ComputeAssignment
│ atm_action? : ATOMIC_ACTION
│ role? : ROLE
│ perms! : ROLE ↔
│              (PERMISSION × ATOMIC_ACTION × RESOURCE)
├──────────────────────────────────────────────────────────
│ perms! = {p : permission; rsrc : resource |
│              (role? ↦ (p, atm_action?, rsrc)) ∈ concrete_Assignment •
│              (role? ↦ (p, atm_action?, rsrc))}
└──────────────────────────────────────────────────────────
```

The following query is a result for the provided action Read and the role Doctor. Jaza tells us that there is one read permission associated to a doctor, named PatientRecord.

```
JAZA> ;FindPermissions
  Input atm\_action? = Read
  Input role? = Doctor
  perms!== {(Doctor, ("PatientRecord", Read, MedicalRecords))}
```

5.5 Finding Duplicate Roles

The schema FindDuplicateRoles allows us to search for duplicate roles. This query is useful to determine whether two roles have the same privileges in a secure system. This schema returns two roles, which are different but are associated with the same sets of atomic actions.

```
┌─ FindDuplicateRoles ─────────────────────────────────────
│ ΞSets ; Ξ ComputeAssignment
│ role1!, role2! : ROLE
│ aSet1!, aSet2! : 𝔽 ATOMIC_ACTION
├──────────────────────────────────────────────────────────
│ role1! ∈ role ∧ role2! ∈ role
│ role1! ≠ role2!
│ aSet1! = {p : permission; a : ATOMIC_ACTION; rsrc : resource |
│              (role1! ↦ (p, a, rsrc)) ∈ concrete_Assignment • a}
│ aSet2! = {p : permission; a : ATOMIC_ACTION; rsrc : resource |
│              (role2! ↦ (p, a, rsrc)) ∈ concrete_Assignment • a}
│ aSet1! = aSet2!
└──────────────────────────────────────────────────────────
```

The following query reports that Patient and EmergencyOfficer are duplicate roles, more precisely they have the permissions to perform the same actions.

```
Jaza ; FindDuplicateRoles
role1!==Patient, role2!==EmergencyOfficer
```

Availability of Data. Utilization of a particular service is handled by availability properties, which are particularly relevant in emergency situations. The availability properties offered by RBAC deal with granting permissions, which will ensure that a resource is available to a user. RBAC aims at avoiding undesirable states in which a user who is entitled to an access permission does not get it. To this end, we propose formal queries, which can be used to review RBAC-based policies. For example, it is significant to determine the minimum information about a patient that can be accessed by everyone. Thus, the availability of operations in our designed policy that could be used in such cases has to be checked.

5.6   Atomic Action Accessed by All

The operation schema AccessAll returns the atomic operations accessible by all roles of a system. The declaration part includes an output variable action!. The given predicate returns the atomic actions accessible by all roles.

$$
\begin{array}{|l}
\_AccessAll _____ \\
\Xi Sets;\ \ \Xi ComputeAssignment \\
action! : ATOMIC\_ACTION \\
\hline
\forall\, r : role \bullet (\exists\, p : permission;\ rsrc : resource \bullet \\
\qquad\qquad (r \mapsto (p, action!, rsrc)) \in concrete\_Assignment) \\
\end{array}
$$

```
Jaza ;AccessAll
action!==Read
```

5.7   Atomic Action Access by Nobody

The operation schema AccessNobody returns the atomic action, which is completely inaccessible by all roles.

$$
\begin{array}{|l}
\_AccessNobody _____ \\
\Xi Sets;\ \ \Xi ComputeAssignment \\
action! : ATOMIC\_ACTION \\
\hline
\forall\, r : role \bullet (\forall\, p : permission;\ rsrc : resource \bullet \\
\qquad\qquad (r \mapsto (p, action!, rsrc)) \notin concrete\_Assignment) \\
\end{array}
$$

It includes an output variable action!, which has the type of an atomic action. The predicate part checks for the inaccessible atomic actions.

```
JAZA> ;AccessNobody
  action!==Create
```

6   Separation of Duty Constraints

Separation of Duty (SoD) constraints are an optional construct of RBAC and are used to address conflicts of interest among roles, which consist of two categories, Static Separation of Duty (SSD) and Dynamic Separation of Duty (DSD).

The SSD takes care of conflicts of interest and ensures that a user does not take some conflicting roles even in different sessions. These constraints are specified over UA assignments as pairs of roles. UA is restricted during sessions. This ensures that if a user is assigned to a role, the user can never take the prohibited role. SSD can be applied not only to colluding users but also to groups, which are collections of users. Permissions can be associated with both users and groups.

DSD is the second kind of constraint offered by RBAC (Fig. 1). These constraints are intended to limit the permissions that are available to a user, whilst SSD constraints reduce the number of potential permissions that can be made available to a user. This is realized by placing constraints on the users that can be assigned to a set of roles. The main difference between SSD and DSD constraints lies in the context in which they are used. SSD are imposed on user's total permission space, but DSD restricts the users to activate the roles within or across a user's sessions. For example, a user Bob may have been assigned with two roles i.e., *Doctor* and *Patient*, but he may not exercise the permissions of both roles in the same session. In the RBAC model, a session is a traditional way of communicating information between a user and a system during a given time interval. Session management in RBAC deals with functions such as session creation for users including role activation/deactivation, enforcing constraints (e.g., DSD) on role activation. An obligatory part of DSD constraints is the use of sessions. In the following, we formally specify SoD constraints using the Z notation.

__ *RoleAssignment* _____

Sets

conflicting_Roles : $ROLE \leftrightarrow ROLE$

role_Assignment : $USER \leftrightarrow ROLE$

_____

dom *conflicting_Roles* $\subseteq$ *role*

ran *conflicting_Roles* $\subseteq$ *role*

dom *role_Assignment* $\subseteq$ *user*

ran *role_Assignment* $\subseteq$ *role*

$\forall\, u : user \bullet (\forall\, i, j : role$

$\qquad | \, ((u \mapsto i) \in role\_Assignment) \land ((u \mapsto j) \in role\_Assignment)$

$\qquad \bullet \, ((i, j) \notin conflicting\_Roles)))$

_____

The declaration in RoleAssignment contains relations describing conflicting roles (conflicting_Roles) and for assigning roles to users (role_Assignment). They are defined as part of the security policy of a system. The first four constraints ensure that the relations to which the schema is applied are actually defined on the roles and users from Sets (cf. Sect. 4.2). The last predicate specifies that any two roles assigned to a user are not from the conflicting roles set.

The subsequent schema SessionRoles formalizes DSD constraints. The schema includes one partial function session_User, because the users of a session have to be considered when checking the role assignment. The relation session_Role assigns roles to sessions, and like in the previous schema, conflicting_Roles_DSD describes the conflicting pairs of roles.

In the predicate part, the constraints for restricting domain and range (similarly to RoleAssignment) have been omitted. The first listed constraint states that whenever a user is assigned to a session with specific roles, the user should have these as pre-assigned roles. The last constraint specifies that the roles taken in one session should not be contained in the set of conflicting roles.

$$
\begin{array}{l}
\rule{3cm}{0pt}\textit{SessionRoles}\rule{6cm}{0pt}\\
\hline
\textit{Sets};\ \textit{RoleAssignment}\\
\textit{session\_User} : \textit{SESSION} \nrightarrow \textit{USER}\\
\textit{session\_Role} : \textit{ROLE} \leftrightarrow \textit{SESSION}\\
\textit{conflicting\_Roles\_DSD} : \textit{ROLE} \leftrightarrow \textit{ROLE}\\
\hline
\vdots\\
\forall\, r : \textit{role} \bullet (\forall\, s : \textit{session}\\
\rule{1.2cm}{0pt}\bullet\ (r, s) \in \textit{session\_Role} \Rightarrow (\textit{session\_User}(s), r) \in \textit{role\_Assignment})\\
\forall\, s : \textit{session} \bullet (\forall\, i, j : \textit{role} \mid ((i, s) \in \textit{session\_Role}) \wedge ((j, s) \in \textit{session\_Role})\\
\rule{1.2cm}{0pt}\bullet\ ((i, j) \notin \textit{conflicting\_Roles\_DSD}))\\
\hline
\end{array}
$$

In the security policy of Fig. 2 let us assume that a doctor is permitted to exercise two roles, i.e., a patient and a doctor. This can be regarded as a serious threat to the medical records where a patient, actually a doctor, compromises the information integrity, because a doctor may perform operations which a patient is not supposed to perform. However, such scenarios are avoidable by introducing an SSD constraint such that a doctor and a patient are specified as conflicting roles. However, this restricts the doctor who might be a patient at some point. In turn, as a solution, we can employ a DSD constraint, which enables exercising both roles but not in one session. Similarly, the role hierarchy (see Fig. 1) can be combined with SSD or DSD to avoid conflicting roles within the hierarchy.

7   Conclusions and Perspectives

This paper presents a formal approach to reviewing healthcare security policies. The proposed approach integrates the Z notation with security design models in order to assess access control rules of an EHR system. The applied idea follows the security-by-design principle and hence exhibits a strategy to cope with internal threats by investigating security properties such as integrity and confidentiality. The Jaza tool is applied to validate formal specifications. Note that in our approach, the formally translated model (the initial state space) does not grow, and it avoids any further complex computations except using the queries to validate the model.

Abundant research literature can be found on how to translate graphical models to formal notations. Nonetheless, to reap out benefits from such formal translations, it is necessary to apply tools and techniques that facilitates easy validation and verification of formal models. Inspired by this, our approach takes such gaps into account. Also, the approach does not require mathematically skilled validation engineers for the following reasons: 1) working with only graphical models of security policies, and 2) automated translation of graphical models besides the reviewing queries. The approach is generic in a sense that it can be used to design and validate other secure information systems irrespective of a particular domain. The paper has only addressed the internal threats (i.e., from the system users). However, UML profiles such as UMLsec [Jür05] can be applied to model and verify systems against external threats.

Currently, the SoD constraints of RBAC are inherently restricted: For instance, a hospital may require an emergency officer to have four roles out of six, but SoD constraints can only be applied over a pair of roles. Our future work includes extending this toolset by overcoming such deficiencies as well as automating the query generation process to help building quality models in the healthcare domain. The tool's performance will also be evaluated using larger models with an extended and complete set of queries.

Acknowledgments. This work has been supported by the projects SAFEHR and GAVES funded by Macao Science and Technology Development Fund, and partly supported by the ANR Selkis Project under grant ANR-08-SEGI-018.

References

[AH07]   Ahn, G.-J., Hu, H.: Towards realizing a formal RBAC model in real systems. In: Lotz, V., Thuraisingham, B.M. (eds.) Proceedings of the 12th ACM Symposium on Access Control Models and Technologies, SACMAT 2007, Sophia Antipolis, France, June 20-22, pp. 215–224. ACM (2007)

[AJ10]   Appari, A., Johnson, M.E.: Information security and privacy in healthcare: current state of research. Int. J. of Internet and Enterprise Management 6(4), 279–314 (2010)

[AK06]   Abdallah, A.E., Khayat, E.J.: Formal Z specifications of several flat role-based access control models. In: 30th Annual IEEE/NASA Software Engineering Workshop (SEW), pp. 282–292. IEEE CS (2006)

[BCDE09] Basin, D.A., Clavel, M., Doser, J., Egea, M.: Automated analysis of security-design models. Information & Software Technology 51(5), 815–831 (2009)

[BL75]   Bell, D., LaPadula, L.: Secure computer system: Unified exposition and multics interpretation. Technical report, MITRE Corp, Bedford (1975)

[Bos95]   Boswell, A.: Specification and validation of a security policy model. IEEE Trans. Software Eng. 21(2), 63–68 (1995)

[Bow03]   Bowen, J.: Formal Specification and Documentation using Z: A Case Study Approach. Thomson Publishing (2003)

[DOD85]   DOD 5200.28-STD. Trusted computer system evaluation criteria. Technical report, United States Department of Defense (1985)

[DW96]   Davies, J., Woodcock, J.: Using Z: Specification, Refinement, and Proof. Prentice Hall (1996) ISBN 0-13-948472-8

[FSG+01]   Ferraiolo, D.F., Sandhu, R., Gavrila, S., Kuhn, D.R., Chandramouli, R.: Proposed NIST standard for role-based access control. ACM Trans. Inf. Syst. Secur. 4(3), 224–274 (2001)

[Hal94]   Hall, A.: Specifying and interpreting class hierarchies in Z. In: Bowen, J.P., Hall, J.A. (eds.) Z User Workshop, pp. 120–138. Springer (1994)

[HY06]   Hasan, R., Yurcik, W.: A statistical analysis of disclosed storage security breaches. In: Proceedings of the 2006 ACM Workshop on Storage Security and Survivability, StorageSS 2006, Alexandria, VA, USA, October 30, pp. 1–8. ACM (2006)

[Jou09]   Rubenstein, S.: Are your medical records at risk? Wall Street Journal (2009)

[Jür05]   Jürjens, J.: Secure systems development with UML. Springer (2005)

[LBD02]   Lodderstedt, T., Basin, D., Doser, J.: SecureUML: A UML-based modeling language for model-driven security. In: Jézéquel, J.-M., Hussmann, H., Cook, S. (eds.) UML 2002. LNCS, vol. 2460, pp. 426–441. Springer, Heidelberg (2002)

[LIM+11]   Ledru, Y., Idani, A., Milhau, J., Qamar, N., Laleau, R., Richier, J.-L., Labiadh, M.-A.: Taking into account functional models in the validation of IS security policies. In: Salinesi, C., Pastor, O. (eds.) CAiSE Workshops 2011. LNBIP, vol. 83, pp. 592–606. Springer, Heidelberg (2011)

[LQI+11]   Ledru, Y., Qamar, N., Idani, A., Richier, J.-L., Labiadh, M.-A.: Validation of security policies by the animation of Z specifications. In: Breu, R., Crampton, J., Lobo, J. (eds.) Proceedings of the 16th ACM Symposium on Access Control Models and Technologies, SACMAT 2011, Innsbruck, Austria, June 15-17, pp. 155–164. ACM (2011)

[MIL+11]   Milhau, J., Idani, A., Laleau, R., Labiadh, M.-A., Ledru, Y., Frappier, M.: Combining UML, ASTD and B for the formal specification of an access control filter. Innov. Syst. Softw. Eng. 7, 303–313 (2011)

[MSGC07]   Morimoto, S., Shigematsu, S., Goto, Y., Cheng, J.: Formal verification of security specifications with common criteria. In: Proceedings of the 2007 ACM Symposium on Applied Computing (SAC), Seoul, Korea, March 11-15, pp. 1506–1512. ACM (2007)

[QLI11]   Qamar, N., Ledru, Y., Idani, A.: Validation of security-design models using Z. In: Qin, S., Qiu, Z. (eds.) ICFEM 2011. LNCS, vol. 6991, pp. 259–274. Springer, Heidelberg (2011)

[SM02]   Schaad, A., Moffett, J.D.: A lightweight approach to specification and analysis of role-based access control extensions. In: Proceedings of the Seventh ACM Symposium on Access Control Models and Technologies, pp. 13–22. ACM (2002)

[Spi92]   Spivey, J.M.: The Z Notation: A Reference Manual, 2nd edn. Prentice Hall International Series in Computer Science (1992)

[TMB06]   Teije, A., Marcos, M., Balser, M., et al.: Improving medical protocols by formal methods. Artif. Intell. Med. 36(3), 193–209 (2006)

[TRA+09]   Toahchoodee, M., Ray, I., Anastasakis, K., Georg, G., Bordbar, B.: En-
           suring spatio-temporal access control for real-world applications. In: Pro-
           ceedings of the 14th ACM Symposium on Access Control Models and
           Technologies, pp. 13–22. ACM, New York (2009)
[YHHZ06]   Yuan, C., He, Y., He, J., Zhou, Z.: A verifiable formal specification for
           RBAC model with constraints of separation of duty. In: Lipmaa, H., Yung,
           M., Lin, D. (eds.) Inscrypt 2006. LNCS, vol. 4318, pp. 196–210. Springer,
           Heidelberg (2006)
[ZWCJ02]   Zao, J., Wee, H., Chu, J., Jackson, D.: RBAC schema verification using
           lightweight formal model and constraint analysis. Technical report, MIT,
           Cambridge (2002)

A Formal Diagrammatic Approach to Compensable Workflow Modelling

Adrian Rutle[1,2], Hao Wang[1], and Wendy MacCaull[1]

[1] Centre for Logic and Information, St. Francis Xavier University, Canada
{hwang,wmaccaul}@stfx.ca
[2] Aalesund University College, Faculty of Engineering and Natural Sciences, Norway
adru@hials.no

Abstract. Workflows consist of interconnected tasks which are executed to achieve predefined business goals. When some tasks fail during execution, compensation can be used as an error-handling procedure to remove side-effects of already finished tasks. This paper extends our formal diagrammatic approach to workflow modelling (which uses principles from model-driven engineering (MDE)) to account for the phenomenon of compensation. Both static semantics, represented by instances of workflow models, and dynamic semantics, represented by a transition system, are described. In MDE, models are first class entities of the development process from which executable application code is generated. The use of MDE technologies is especially important for software in health services delivery where processes are safety critical, highly localised and frequently change.

1 Introduction

Workflow software systems improve productivity and quality of service; however, defects in a workflow model may have severe consequences. While business modelling facilitates involvement of domain experts and business managers in the modelling phase of workflow software development, a formal foundation is needed to guarantee that workflow models are correct and represent the intended system. Currently there is still a gap between practice (programming) and theory (formal methods and analysis techniques) [16]. For example, the widely used Business Process Model and Notation (BPMN) [19] is a diagrammatic language for business process modelling, which is designed as a standard notation readily understandable by various participants with different expertise due to its graphical nature [20]. Because Business Process Execution Language for Web Services (BPEL4WS) [17] is currently the de facto standard for business process execution, there are several attempts to translate the models in BPMN to BPEL4WS. However, it has been found that the two languages are fundamentally different, thus translation can be applied only to a subset of BPMN [21]. A more serious problem is that changes in BPEL4WS implementation are difficult to synchronise with the BPMN model. In healthcare software systems, changes in software to account for customisation to local settings and updates of protocols are frequent and inevitable.

Distributed and heterogeneous business processes make business transactions long lasting, the so-called *Long-Running Transactions* (LRT) [7,8]. Traditional all-or-nothing atomicity is no longer appropriate for these transactions because it is impractical to lock

J. Weber and I. Perseil (Eds.): FHIES 2012, LNCS 7789, pp. 194–212, 2013.

resources for a long period of time and some activities may be interactive, hence cannot be easily check-pointed [7]. Therefore, a relaxed notion of atomicity called *compensation* is used. In compensable workflow modelling, each task is combined with a compensation task. When a failure occurs during the execution of the workflow, the compensation tasks related to the already finished tasks are activated to remove side-effects and restore the system to a desired state. Note that compensation is not equivalent to undoing, e.g., the damages caused to a patient by a failed procedure cannot be undone; in that situation other arrangements for mitigation are required.

There are efforts towards developing rigorous formal methods, especially process calculi, for specification and analysis of concurrent, distributed and mobile systems. Although various process calculi have been proposed, addressing some aspects of workflow executions, most domain experts, software engineers and workflow model designers are unable to use them due to their complexity.

In previous work [25,27], we proposed a model-driven engineering (MDE) approach to business process modelling, combining the best of the two worlds: a visually appealing language making modelling easier and a formal foundation facilitating automatic software generation and verification. In this paper, we extend our approach by adding support for compensation. The formal approach we use is based on the Diagram Predicate Framework (DPF) [10,11,24,26] which provides a formalisation of (meta)modelling and model transformations based on category theory [4] and graph transformations [12]. In [25,27], we extended the formal foundation of DPF to define semantics for workflow models, defining the dynamic semantics of models by a transition system where the states are instances and the transition relations are described by applications of transformation rules. Here we augment the workflow models by combining each task with a compensation task and define the static and dynamic semantics accordingly. We also discuss a method to ensure the soundness [2] of workflow models.

Unlike traditional approaches where models are used merely for documentation purposes, MDE employs models as the primary artefacts of the software development process. In this way, the relation between the final result of the development process – the executable software system – and the workflow models remains intact during software development, maintenance, deployment, etc. In our approach, each state of the workflow software system corresponds to an instance of the workflow model, and each execution path allowed by the system corresponds to a sequence of instance transitions. This correspondence, one of the main advantages of our MDE-based approach, facilitates the use of verification, analysis and simulation techniques on models, ensuring that the analysis results are valid for the software system.

MDE technologies are especially valuable when applied to workflow for safety critical systems such as those involved in health care. Health care protocols are often complex, and are usually based on clinical guidelines written in natural language. These guidelines must be general enough to fit the variations that arise from local settings – whether they be a hospital, a doctor's office, a clinic, etc. Updates of guidelines are frequent to reflect advances in knowledge and treatments. The complexity of some guidelines results in inconsistencies and/or ambiguities. Yet conformance to guidelines is essential to the health of the patient. Following the MDE approach, we abstract the protocols through modelling, which helps the domain experts (clinicians) clarify meaning and provides them with an opportunity to deal with the inconsistencies and ambiguities that may arise. Behavioural anomalies (errors) in these models, not obvious by inspection of the models, can be found through the use of formal verification and other analysis techniques – before the protocols are used on patients. MDE facilitates the generation of (correct) code from the models. Customisations and adaptations of the protocol occur at the model level, not at the code level, so compliance with the protocol can be ensured in the many customisations and updates that are inevitable for healthcare protocols. An implemented workflow software system, which reflects the requirements of the model, and which can be used to guide and direct the entire care team on the process they are to follow, is the final desired result. Overall, the MDE approach has the potential to provide executable software which can ensure conformance with healthcare protocols, which, as an end result, enhances the health and safety of the patient.

The remainder of the paper is structured as follows. Section 2 outlines the metamodelling approach and reviews our formal, diagrammatic approach to workflow modelling. Section 3 introduces the main contributions of the paper: our approach to compensable workflow modelling and some analysis techniques to check soundness of compensable workflow models. In Section 4, some related work is discussed. Finally, Section 5 concludes and presents some ideas for future work.

2   Metamodelling and Modelling Languages

Using the MDE methodology, a workflow modelling language is described by a metamodel, from which a corresponding model editor is constructed. The metamodel defines the abstract syntax of the modelling language; i.e., it defines the types and relations between types, whereas the model editor is used to create and modify workflow models. Each workflow model must conform to the language's metamodel; i.e., it must respect the typing and other constraints of the language. For example, Fig. 1 shows a metamodel with the *concepts* Task and Flow. The model editor constructed from this metamodel will allow users to define workflow models consisting of specific tasks and flows, e.g., Check eligibility and f, respectively.

The model editor must deal with two kinds of constraints. First, *metamodel constraints*; that is, if there are constraints *added to* the metamodel, the editor should not allow definition of models which violate these constraints. For example, if in the metamodel we require that flows are (transitively) irreflexive (see Fig. 1) the model editor should not allow users to define loops in workflow models. Second, *model constraints*; that is, if users want to define models with a satisfactory degree of precision, they sometimes need to add constraints to the models defined by the model editor. Examples of this kind of constraint are routing constraints such as XOR, AND, OR, etc.

The first kind of constraint is usually enforced by developing internal mechanisms when the model editor is constructed from the metamodel; this prevents the definition of models which do not *conform to* the language's metamodel, in the sense which we will make precise below. The second kind of constraint may be formulated by adding predicates on the structure of the models; e.g., [exactly-one,c] for an XOR constraint which has a condition c (see Fig. 1). This constraint describes some property of the workflow model; e.g. in the figure, it defines that exactly one of the two flows f or g can be followed, based on the eligibility condition. Obviously, this property must

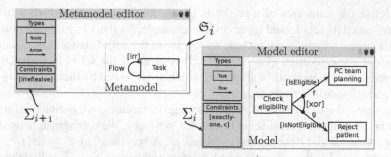

Fig. 1. A metamodel and a model editor, and correspondence with a modelling formalism $\mathcal{F}_i = (\Sigma_i, \mathfrak{S}_i, \Sigma_{i+1})$

be encoded in the software system which will be generated from the model. And most importantly with regard to MDE, to enable reasoning about models – i.e., before code-generation – the semantics of these properties must be already well-defined in the modelling language. For models, the semantics is all about which structures are qualified as their instances; that is, the same way as a metamodel defines certain restrictions or language requirements which each model conforming to the metamodel must satisfy, a model defines certain domain requirements which each instance conforming to the model must satisfy.

Thus to understand how a software system generated from a model will behave, it is necessary to inspect the instances of the model. For models describing system structure, such as data models, this means that the modelling environment should facilitate instantiation of models, i.e., creation of instances of models. For models describing system behaviour, such as workflow models, this means that the modelling environment should facilitate, in addition to instantiation of models, transition of instances, i.e., creation of execution paths. In fact, constructing an instance editor from a model is not different from constructing a model editor from a metamodel since a metamodel is a model with the role of being a metamodel wrt. models defined by the corresponding model editor. Like many metamodelling frameworks, DPF supports seamless definition of (meta)model editors from (meta)models. We have extended DPF with the necessary techniques to support time and the creation of execution paths in [25,27]; this paper adds support for compensation in workflow modelling.

Now we briefly review the basic concepts of DPF which we use for the formalisation of workflow modelling; for details and formal definitions, the interested reader can consult [24,26]. In DPF, a model is represented by a *specification* $\mathfrak{S}$. A specification (or a model) $\mathfrak{S} = (S, C^{\mathfrak{S}} : \Sigma)$ consists of an *underlying graph* S together with a set of *constraints* $C^{\mathfrak{S}}$ which are specified by means of a *predicate signature* Σ. A predicate signature consists of a collection of *predicates*, each having a name and an arity (or shape graph). A constraint consists of a predicate from the signature together with the subgraph of the model's underlying graph which is affected by the constraint; e.g., a constraint in the model in Fig. 1 consists of [exactly-one, c] and a subgraph of the model which in this case is the whole underlying graph of the model. A specification morphism is a constraint preserving graph homomorphism [12] between the underlying graphs of the specifications. We will use the terms "specification" and "model" interchangeably.

We define the semantics of a predicate as the set of all graphs which satisfy the predicate, called its set of valid instances. For example, for the [irreflexive] predicate all graphs which do not include a loop are in the set of its valid instances. The semantics of a specification $\mathfrak{S} = (S, C^{\mathfrak{S}} : \Sigma)$ is given by the set of its instances. The set of instances of $\mathfrak{S}$ consists of all graphs which are (i) typed by the underlying graph S of $\mathfrak{S}$ and (ii) satisfy the constraints $C^{\mathfrak{S}}$ of $\mathfrak{S}$.

To facilitate the discussion of metamodelling hierarchies, we define conformance relation between models at adjacent levels of a hierarchy. We distinguish between two kinds of conformance: *typed by* and *conforms to*. A specification $\mathfrak{S} = (S, C^{\mathfrak{S}} : \Sigma)$ is typed by a graph T if there exists a graph homomorphism $\iota : S \to T$, called the *typing morphism*, while $\mathfrak{S}$ is said to conform to a specification $\mathfrak{T} = (T, C^{\mathfrak{T}} : \Sigma)$ if $\mathfrak{S}$ is typed by T and S is an instance of $\mathfrak{T}$; e.g., if we add a flow f' from the task Check eligibility to itself in Fig. 1; then the model would still be typed by the metamodel, however, it would not conform to it because of the violation of the irreflexivity constraint. We define typed specification morphisms as specification morphisms which preserve typing.

In DPF, a modelling language is described by a modelling formalism $\mathcal{F}_i = (\Sigma_i, \mathfrak{S}_i, \Sigma_{i+1})$. Fig. 1 shows the correspondence between the elements of modelling formalisms and modelling languages. The corresponding metamodel of the modelling language is represented by the specification $\mathfrak{S}_i$ which has its constraints (e.g. [irreflexive]) formulated by predicates from the signature Σ_{i+1}. These constraints of $\mathfrak{S}_i$ should be satisfied by all specifications, $\mathfrak{S}_{i-1} = (S_{i-1}, C^{\mathfrak{S}_{i-1}} : \Sigma_i)$, which are specified by $\mathcal{F}_i$. The constructs which are used to define constraints at the next level (e.g. [exactly-one, c]) are located in the signature Σ_i. As we see from the figure, there is no difference between metamodel editors and model editors.

2.1 Workflow Modelling

We now develop a formal, conceptual framework for modelling compensable health workflows. Workflow modelling languages provide constructs to define tasks and their routing flows. Fig. 2 shows a modelling formalism $\mathcal{F}_2 = (\Sigma_2, \mathfrak{S}_2, \Sigma_3)$ used for the specification of workflow models, with a metamodel defining the types Task and Flow, and a signature containing predicates for splitting and merging. The figure shows only parts of Σ_2, Σ_1 and $\mathfrak{S}_1$; the details are shown in Tables 1 and 2 and Fig. 3, respectively.

Table 1 shows signature Σ_2 with some predicates which are useful for workflow modelling. The predicates have spans or sinks of two arrows as arity, and are used to define relations between different flows. We could define these predicates with arities being spans or sinks of any finite number of arrows, however two arrows suffice to explain the modelling formalism. The predicate [exactly-one, c] is used to indicate that exactly one of the two flows must be followed; the predicate [all-premises] is used to indicate that both flows f and g must be followed to start running the task Y. The predicate [exactlyone, c] has a parameter condition c, which is a proposition that may evaluate to true or false, or it may not be evaluated yet. As seen from the table, for the predicate [exactly-one, c], one of the flows will have c as a condition, the other one will have the negation of c; thus forcing exactly one flow to be followed. To save space, we omit from Table 1 the other usual predicates used in workflow modelling, such as [at-least-one, c_1, c_2] and [exactly-one-premise].

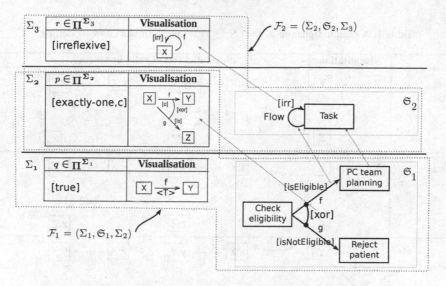

Fig. 2. Two modelling formalisms $\mathcal{F}_2 = (\Sigma_2, \mathfrak{S}_2, \Sigma_3)$ and $\mathcal{F}_1 = (\Sigma_1, \mathfrak{S}_1, \Sigma_2)$ for creation of workflow models and instances of workflow models, respectively

The semantics of the predicates in Table 1 is formulated by enumerating the set of their valid instances. We use x:X to denote the typing morphism $\iota : x \rightarrow X$, and we write :X if x is unique. We have used $\boxed{\text{x:X}}^{<D|E|R|F>}$ to denote the case where we have one of the following: $\boxed{\text{x:X}}^{<D>}$, $\boxed{\text{x:X}}^{<E>}$, $\boxed{\text{x:X}}^{<R>}$ or $\boxed{\text{x:X}}^{<F>}$. Later it will be clear that <D>, <E>, <R>, <F>, <⊤>, <⊥> and <?> are visualisations for the predicates [disabled], [enabled], [running], [finished], [true], [false] and [not-evaluated], respectively, of the signature Σ_1 in Table 2. These predicates are used to annotate task and flow instances with their individual execution states.

As we see from Table 1, the semantics of – i.e., the set of valid instances of – the predicates of the signature Σ_2 is explained in terms of graphs annotated by predicates from the signature Σ_1. In other words, the set of valid instances does not consist of graphs, but consists of specifications which have their constraints formulated by means of predicates from the signature Σ_1. This semantic dependence is necessary since, in order to define meaningful semantics for predicates like [exactly-one, c], we need to consider the execution states (such as disabled, enabled, etc.) of the task instances x:X, y:Y and z:Z. These execution states belong to the instances of workflow models, and they are indicated by predicates from the signature Σ_1, such as [disabled], [enabled], etc. The details of the static and dynamic semantics of our workflow models are given in Section 2.2; first we show an example from the health care domain.

Fig. 3 shows a simplified version of a Palliative Care (PC) team building workflow model, which details $\mathfrak{S}_1$ that is specified by $\mathcal{F}_2$ and used as the metamodel of $\mathcal{F}_1$ in Fig. 2. The specification $\mathfrak{S}_1$ captures the following requirements:

R1 Patient's eligibility has to be checked first *before* any other tasks are performed;
R2 *If* patient is eligible for PC, build PC team;
R3 *If* patient is not eligible for PC, reject patient;

Table 1. A sample signature $\Sigma_2 = (\Pi^{\Sigma_2}, \alpha^{\Sigma_2})$ used for workflow modelling

p	Visualisation	Semantics (set of valid instances)
[exactly-one, c]	X $\xrightarrow{\ f\ }$ Y, $[c]$, $[xor]$, $[!c]$, g → Z	$<$D$|$E$|$R$|$F$>$ x:X $\xrightarrow[<?>]{:f}$ y:Y$^{<D>}$:g $<?>$ → z:Z$^{<D>}$ $<$F$>$ x:X $\xrightarrow[<\top>]{:f}$ y:Y$^{<E|R|F>}$:g $<\bot>$ → z:Z$^{<D>}$
[all-together]	X $\xrightarrow{\ f\ }$ Y, $[and]$, g → Z	$<$D$|$E$|$R$|$F$>$ x:X $\xrightarrow{:f}$ y:Y$^{<D>}$:g → z:Z$^{<D>}$ $<$F$>$ x:X $\xrightarrow{:f}$ y:Y$^{<E|R|F>}$:g → z:Z$^{<E|R|F>}$
[all-premises]	X $\xrightarrow{\ f\ }$ Y, $[and']$, Z $\xrightarrow{g}$	$<$D$|$E$|$R$|$F$>$ x:X $\xrightarrow{:f}$ y:Y$^{<D>}$ $<$D$|$E$|$R$|$F$>$ z:Z $\xrightarrow{:g}$ $<$F$>$ x:X $\xrightarrow{:f}$ y:Y$^{<E|R|F>}$ $<$F$>$ z:Z $\xrightarrow{:g}$
[at-least-one-premise]	X $\xrightarrow{\ f\ }$ Y, $[or']$, Z $\xrightarrow{g}$	$<$D$|$E$|$R$|$F$>$ x:X $\xrightarrow{:f}$ y:Y$^{<D>}$ $<$D$|$E$|$R$|$F$>$ z:Z $\xrightarrow{:g}$ $<$F$>$ x:X $\xrightarrow{:f}$ y:Y$^{<E|R|F>}$ $<$D$|$E$|$R$|$F$>$ z:Z $\xrightarrow{:g}$

R4 A patient is *either* eligible *or* not eligible for PC, but not both;

R5 *After* PC team planning, assign *both* general practitioner (GP) *and* PC nurse;

R6 *If both* GP and PC nurse are assigned, submit the team information.

In $\mathfrak{S}_1$, R1 is specified by the task Check Eligibility which is the only task with no incoming flows. R2, R3 and R4 are specified by the tasks PC team planning and Reject patient, the two flows f and g, and the constraint [exactly-one, $isEligible$]. R5 is specified by the tasks Assign GP and Assign PC nurse, and the flows i and j with the constraint [all-together]. R6 is specified by the task Submit team info and the flows i' and j', and the constraint [all-premises].

2.2 Semantics of Workflow Models

Recall that the *static semantics* of a workflow model $\mathfrak{S}_1$ is given by the set of its instances. These instances represent discrete, static states of the workflow software system developed from the workflow model. We defined the set of instances of a model $\mathfrak{S}$ to consist of graphs that are typed by the underlying graph of $\mathfrak{S}$ and that satisfy the constraints of $\mathfrak{S}$. In this section, we define the set of instances to be a set of specifications $\mathfrak{S}_0 = (S_0, C^{\mathfrak{S}_0}: \Sigma_1)$ rather than graphs. This is because Σ_2 is semantically dependent on Σ_1; which means that the set of valid instances of predicates of Σ_2 consists of

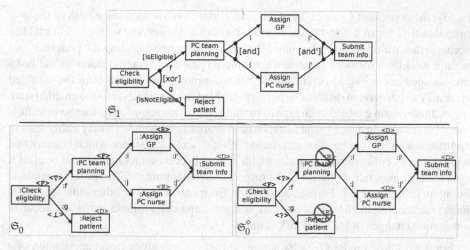

Fig. 3. The specification $\mathfrak{S}_1$ and two sample specifications $\mathfrak{S}_0$ and $\mathfrak{S}_0^\diamond$, where only $\mathfrak{S}_0$ is an instance of $\mathfrak{S}_1$; the instance editor would prevent creation of $\mathfrak{S}_0^\diamond$

specifications rather than graphs. We define a modelling formalism $\mathcal{F}_1 = (\Sigma_1, \mathfrak{S}_1, \Sigma_2)$ which enables us to create instances $\mathfrak{S}_0$ of a workflow model $\mathfrak{S}_1$ (see Figs. 2 and 3).

At any state of the workflow software system, task instances, e.g., :Check eligibility in $\mathfrak{S}_0$ in Fig. 3, are either *disabled, enabled, running or finished*, according to the constraints specified in the workflow model $\mathfrak{S}_1$. We use the signature Σ_1 shown in Table 2 to annotate task instances in $\mathfrak{S}_0$ accordingly. Moreover, the condition of the predicate [exactly-one, c] may be waiting for evaluation, or be evaluated to either true or false; the signature Σ_1 also includes predicates to annotate flow instances in $\mathfrak{S}_0$ accordingly. The signature Σ_1 has no semantic counterpart since for this modelling environment instances of $\mathfrak{S}_0$ do not have any practical meaning. For this reason, we write "annotations" (instead of "constraints") added to a specification $\mathfrak{S}_0$. Note that states of an individual task instance, e.g., disabled, enabled, etc., should be distinguished from the overall state of a workflow model, which corresponds to a workflow instance.

Fig. 3 shows a specification $\mathfrak{S}_0$ which is specified by $\mathcal{F}_1$ and is an instance of $\mathfrak{S}_1$. In $\mathfrak{S}_0$ the task instance :Assign GP is running (annotated with <R>), the task instance :Assign PC nurse is enabled (annotated with <E>), and the rest of the task instances are either finished or disabled (annotated with <F> and <D>, respectively). The figure also shows a specification $\mathfrak{S}_0^\diamond$ which is not an instance of $\mathfrak{S}_1$. Although $\mathfrak{S}_0^\diamond$ is typed

Table 2. A signature Σ_1 used for annotation of workflow instances

$q \in \Pi^{\Sigma_1}$	Visualisation	$q \in \Pi^{\Sigma_1}$	Visualisation
[enabled]	X <E>	[true]	X $\xrightarrow[\text{<T>}]{\text{f}}$ Y
[disabled]	X <D>	[false]	X $\xrightarrow[\text{<}\perp\text{>}]{\text{f}}$ Y
[running]	X <R>	[not-evaluated]	X $\xrightarrow[\text{<?>}]{\text{f}}$ Y
[finished]	X <F>		

by $\mathfrak{S}_1$, the constraint [exactly-one, $isEligible$] is violated since both of the task instances :PC team planning and :Reject patient are annotated with <E>. In real life scenario this would mean both doing PC team planning and rejecting the patient.

In a workflow software system, when time passes the execution states of the tasks are changed according to certain rules. For example, a task which is in the disabled state may either remain disabled or become enabled; a task which is in the enabled state may either remain enabled or change to running, etc. Correspondingly, for the workflow model $\mathfrak{S}_1$, a task instance (in an instance of $\mathfrak{S}_1$) annotated with <D> may either remain annotated with <D> or become annotated with <E>; a task instance which is annotated with <E> may either remain annotated with <E> or become annotated with <R>, etc. Of course, these annotation changes must respect the constraints in $\mathfrak{S}_1$ in order to continue being an instance of $\mathfrak{S}_1$. Further, a transition from one state to another must include at least one annotation change of one task instance, and cannot include two consecutive annotation changes of the same task instance.

For a workflow model $\mathfrak{S}_1$, a transition $\mathfrak{S}_0 \stackrel{<t>}{\Rightarrow} \mathfrak{S}_0'$ is given by an application of a transformation rule t, where both specifications $\mathfrak{S}_0, \mathfrak{S}_0'$ are instances of $\mathfrak{S}_1$. A transformation rule $t = \mathfrak{L} \stackrel{l}{\hookleftarrow} \mathfrak{K} \stackrel{r}{\hookrightarrow} \mathfrak{R}$ consists of three specifications $\mathfrak{L}, \mathfrak{K}$ and $\mathfrak{R}$, and two inclusion specification morphisms l, r. $\mathfrak{L}$ and $\mathfrak{R}$ are the *left-hand side* (LHS) and *right-hand side* (RHS) of the transformation rule, respectively, while $\mathfrak{K}$ is their interface. $\mathfrak{L} \setminus \mathfrak{K}$ describes the part of a specification which is to be deleted, $\mathfrak{R} \setminus \mathfrak{K}$ describes the part to be added, and $\mathfrak{K}$ describes the overlap between $\mathfrak{L}$ and $\mathfrak{R}$. To save space we omit the technical details of transformation rules, full details may be found in [12,26].

By defining the notions of states and transitions between states we obtain a transition system which we use to provide the dynamic semantics for workflow models. In general, given a set of transformation rules $TR := \{t_1, t_2, ..., t_n\}$, different sequences of rule applications to a start specification may result in different target specifications. A transition system consists of all possible ways of applying the rules from TR to a start specification $\mathfrak{S}$; i.e., it represents all specification transformations $\mathfrak{S} \stackrel{*}{\Rightarrow} \mathfrak{S}'$, $\mathfrak{S} \stackrel{*}{\Rightarrow} \mathfrak{S}''$, ... Below we detail the notion of start specification, but first we show in Table 3 the transformation rules comprising our transition system.

We will explain briefly the general pattern of the rules in Table 3. Rule t_1 is used to change the annotation of a task instance y to <E> when the preceding task instance x is finished. Rules t_2 and t_3 are for changing annotations of task instances from <E> to <R> and from <R> to <F>, respectively. Rules t_4 and t_5 are used to describe the transitions of spans of flow instances, and t_6 and t_7 are used to describe the transitions of sinks of flow instances. The LHSs of t_4 and t_5 are equal, meaning that at any situation when a match of these rules is found, the system may proceed non-deterministically to either of the two states indicated by the RHSs of the rules. That is, either both of the task instances y and z become annotated with <E> or one of them becomes annotated with <E>. These choices define the semantics for splitting with [exactly-one, c], [all-together] and [at-least-one]. Recall that applying the rules must always produce valid instances of the workflow model. If the structure in the workflow model by which x, y, z, f and g are typed is constrained with [all-together], only t_4 will produce a valid instance, and thus only t_4 will be applicable. Analogously, in case of [exactly-one, c] only t_5 is applicable, while in case of [at-least-one] both t_4 and t_5 are applicable. In t_7, one may proceed and enable y although z is not yet finished. This sort of behaviour is necessary for flows which are constrained by [at-least-one-premise]. To save space we have omitted the duals of the rules t_5/t_7 where z is enabled/finished, respectively.

Transition systems in general may be or may not be terminating [12,24]. That is, starting with $\mathfrak{S}$, it may always be possible to apply more rules from *TR*. To achieve termination of our transition system, we control the application of transformation rules through (i) priorities, (ii) the use of *negative application conditions* (NACs) [12] and (iii) requiring that each rule application must result in a specification which conforms to a certain meta-specification. We require that in Table 3 the LHSs of all rules from t_4 to t_7 are NACs for t_1. Informally, this forbids changing the annotation on a single task instance if it is part of a bigger structure. This priority definition is necessary since in a bigger structure there may be dependencies between flow and task instances.

Table 3. Some transformation rules $t = \mathfrak{L} \hookleftarrow \mathfrak{K} \hookrightarrow \mathfrak{R}$ of our transition system

t	$\mathfrak{L}$	$\mathfrak{K}$	$\mathfrak{R}$
t_1	<F>x —a→ y<D>	<F>x —a→ y	<F>x —a→ y<E>
t_2	x<E>	x	x<R>
t_3	x<R>	x	x<F>
t_4	<F>x —a→ y<D> ; x —b→ z<D>	<F>x —a→ y ; x —b→ z	<F>x —a→ y<E> ; x —b→ z<E>
t_5	<F>x —a→ y<D> ; x —b→ z<D>	<F>x —a→ y ; x —b→ z<D>	<F>x —a→ y<E> ; x —b→ z<D>
t_6	<F>x —a→ y<D> ; <F>z —b→	<F>x —a→ y ; <F>z —b→	<F>x —a→ y<E> ; <F>z —b→
t_7	<F>x —a→ y<D> ; <D|E|R>z —b→	<F>x —a→ y ; <D|E|R>z —b→	<F>x —a→ y<E> ; <D|E|R>z —b→

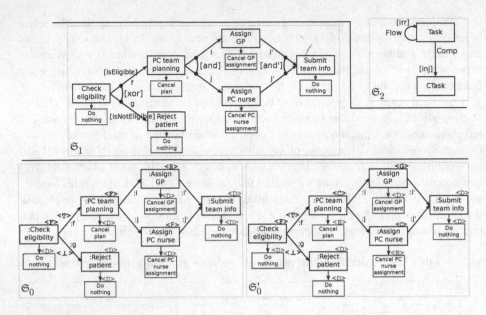

Fig. 4. Metamodelling hierarchy with compensation

3 Compensation and Analysis

In our approach to compensation we combine each task t with a *compensation task* ct, and when a failure occurs after t has finished, the compensation task ct will be executed to remove possible side-effects caused by executing t. We assume that t is atomic in the sense that if it fails during execution, it does not leave any side-effects. Thus only when t is finished it leaves side-effects. To facilitate this, we extend the metamodel $\mathfrak{S}_2$ by adding the new types CTask and Comp (abbreviations for CompensationTask and Compensation), where Comp connects Task to CTask (see $\mathfrak{S}_2$ in Fig. 4). This enforces that in all workflow models $\mathfrak{S}_1$ specified by $\mathcal{F}_2$, whenever a task T:Task is specified, a compensation task cT:CTask and a compensation arrow T:Task $\xrightarrow{\text{co:comp}}$ cT:CTask must also be specified. Moreover, we add a constraint [injection] on Comp (visualised as [inj]), which enforces that two different tasks are not allowed to be connected to the same compensation task. The specification $\mathfrak{S}_1$ in Fig. 4 is an example compensable workflow model which conforms to the extended metamodel $\mathfrak{S}_2$.

Although the formal foundation of the proposed compensable workflow modelling language forces the definition of an additional node for each "normal" task, language designers may choose different visualisations for the combination of tasks and their corresponding compensation tasks, see Fig. 5 for an example. Here we only focus on the formal foundations independent of visualisation effects. In Fig. 5 we ignore neutral compensation tasks which are called Do Nothing. Remark that this is just a visualisation effect and the underlying semantic model will be $\mathfrak{S}_1$ as shown in Fig. 4.

In order to define the static and dynamic semantics for workflow models with compensation, we will also extend the signature Σ_1 with two new predicates, and the

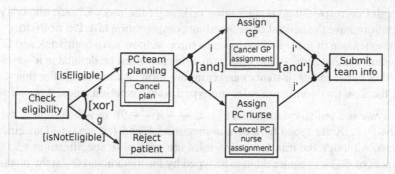

Fig. 5. Possible visualisation of compensation tasks

transition system with five new rules shown in Table 4. The predicate [error] (visualised <G>) is used to annotate a task instance indicating that it has failed. The predicate [compensate] (visualised <C>) is used to annotate a task instance indicating one of the following situations (see Fig. 6): it is under compensation (if the corresponding compensation task is either annotated with <E> or <R>), or it is compensated successfully (if the corresponding compensation task is annotated with <F>), or its compensation also has failed (if the corresponding compensation task is annotated with <G>).

Some restrictions apply when using the two new predicates. First, the predicate [compensate] is only allowed to annotate task instances, since, compensation task instances do not have compensation; i.e., they either finish successfully or fail. Second, only when a task instance is annotated with <C>, is its corresponding compensation task instance allowed to be annotated with <E>, <R>, <F> or <G>, since, as long as a task instance is not under compensation, its corresponding compensation task instance must be disabled. Fig. 6 illustrates these restrictions by showing the allowable combinations.

Fig. 4 shows a compensable workflow model corresponding to $\mathfrak{S}_1$ in Fig. 3 which conforms to the extended metamodel. The figure also shows two instances $\mathfrak{S}_0$ and $\mathfrak{S}_0'$ of $\mathfrak{S}_1$. In $\mathfrak{S}_0$ the task instance :Assign GP is running, but if it fails, as indicated in $\mathfrak{S}_0'$, the task instances :PC team planning and :Assign PC nurse will be notified to start compensation. Note that the corresponding compensation task instance :Cancel GP assignment will not be enabled in this case since the task instance :Assign GP did not finish and hence did not leave any side-effects. Moreover, not every task in $\mathfrak{S}_1$ has

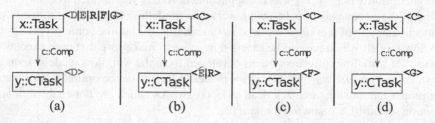

Fig. 6. Allowed combinations of annotations: (a) y is disabled, (b) x is under compensation, (c) x is successfully compensated (d) the compensation y of x has failed

a meaningful corresponding compensation task; e.g., the tasks Check eligibility and Reject patient have the neutral corresponding compensation task Do nothing.

For the extension of the transition system, since we now have both Task and CTask in the metamodel $\mathfrak{S}_2$, some of the transformation rules must be defined in a way which distinguishes between task instances and compensation task instances. For this reason, some of the new transformation rules are typed transformation rules. A *typed trans-formation rule* is a transformation rule $t = \mathfrak{L} \xleftarrow{l} \mathfrak{K} \xrightarrow{r} \mathfrak{R}$ in which each of the specifications $\mathfrak{L}, \mathfrak{K}, \mathfrak{R}$ are typed by a certain metamodel, and l, r are typed specification morphisms. Although the transformation rules are applied to specifications $\mathfrak{S}_0$ which are instances of $\mathfrak{S}_1$, we require them to be typed by the metamodel $\mathfrak{S}_2$ at the meta-level rather than to $\mathfrak{S}_1$. This is because we only need to distinguish between task instances and compensation task instances, and this information is available in the metamodel. In this way, we can define generic transformation rules which are independent of the details of a specific workflow model $\mathfrak{S}_1$. Thus, instead of writing x:aTask:Task in our transformation rules, we write x::Task denoting that the *type of the type* of x is Task.

The new transformation rules are shown in Table 4. Rule t_8 adds the possibility of failure to running (compensation) task instances. Rule t_9 forces the preceding task instance x1 to enable its compensation task instance y1 when the task instance x2 fails. Rule t_{10} forces the task instance x1 to enable its compensation task instance y1 when the compensation task instance y2 of the successor task instance x2 finishes. The rules t_{11} and t_{12} are used to notify other possible parallel branches to start compensation. t_{11} forces every task instance which is enabled or running to fail (or abort), while t_{12} forces every task instance which is finished and is not followed by another finished, compensating or failed task instance, to start compensation. The NAC of t_{12} forbids some application of the rule since we want to force start the compensation of the *last* finished task instance in all parallel branches. This is because, for <F>, the rule should be applied to the last finished task, then rule t_{10} can be used to start compensation of x2. In the case of <C>, it means that x3 has started compensation and x2 will eventually get compensated when x3's compensation is finished successfully. In the case of <G>, finally, it means that the rule t_9 will be used. Rules t_1 through t_8 from Tables 3 and 4 are not typed hence are applicable to both task and compensation task instances.

We can now give a complete control structure of the rules in Tables 3 and 4. In addition to the NAC of rule t_{12} and the restriction that LHSs of all rules t_4 to t_7 are NACs for the rule t_1, we require the highest priority for t_{11}, t_{12}. In Fig. 4 the sequence of transitions t_8, t_{12}, t_9 has happened to transform $\mathfrak{S}_0$ to $\mathfrak{S}_0'$. Remark that although t_{12} has higher priority than t_8, t_{12} was not applicable before t_8 was applied to $\mathfrak{S}_0$.

One of the advantages of formalising workflow modelling languages is to facilitate automatic analysis of workflow models. In this section we outline some properties of workflow models which have to be satisfied in order to make sure that each execution scenario (of workflow software systems developed from the workflow models) *terminates* in an *appropriate* way [1]. Workflow models which have the option to terminate, have proper termination, and lack dead tasks (i.e., tasks which are not enabled in any execution scenario), are said to be *sound* [2].

Since our transition system is based on graph transformations, we use the termination property from graph transformations [12]. More precisely, we have defined our

Table 4. The transformation rules $t = \mathfrak{L} \hookleftarrow \mathfrak{K} \hookrightarrow \mathfrak{R}$ for handling compensation

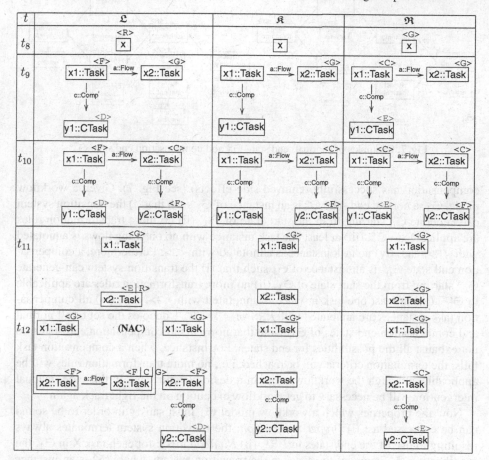

transformation rules in such a way that for any start state of a workflow model, we can guarantee that the transition system will eventually terminate and produce an end state; termination in this sense means that no more transformation rules are applicable. Proving that the transformation rules from Tables 3 and 4 together with the control structures are terminating is straightforward, but outside the scope of this paper. In addition to the termination property of the transition system, we need also to require that each task will be annotated with <E> at least in one state.

First we define start state. Given a workflow model $\mathfrak{S}_1$, start state $\mathfrak{S}_0^s$ is an instance of $\mathfrak{S}_1$ such that the transition system can generate all other specifications starting from $\mathfrak{S}_0^s$, which are instances of $\mathfrak{S}_1$, and, all its task instances with no incoming flows are annotated with <E> and all other task instances are annotated with <D>.

We distinguish between two disjoint sets of end states: *normal end states* (no task instance has failed) and *compensation end states* (some task instances have failed and

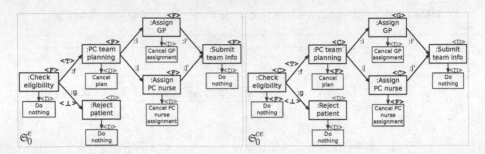

Fig. 7. Examples of (normal) end state $\mathfrak{S}_0^e$ and compensation end state $\mathfrak{S}_0^{ce}$

compensation has successfully removed side-effects) (see Fig. 7). Given a workflow model $\mathfrak{S}_1$, a normal end state $\mathfrak{S}_0^e$ is an instance of $\mathfrak{S}_1$ such that (i) the transition system can generate $\mathfrak{S}_0^e$ starting from the start state of $\mathfrak{S}_1$, (ii) no more transformation rules are applicable to $\mathfrak{S}_0^e$, (iii) at least one task instance with no outgoing flows is annotated with <F>, and, (iv) no task instance is annotated with <G>. Furthermore, a compensation end state $\mathfrak{S}_0^{ce}$ is an instance of $\mathfrak{S}_1$ such that (i) the transition system can generate $\mathfrak{S}_0^{ce}$ starting from the start state of $\mathfrak{S}_1$, (ii) no more transformation rules are applicable to $\mathfrak{S}_0^{ce}$, (iii) at least one task instance is annotated with <G>, and, (iv) all compensation task instances are annotated with <F> or <D>. $E^{\mathfrak{S}_1}$ denotes the set of all normal and compensation end states of $\mathfrak{S}_1$. Note that normal and compensation end states do not exhaust all the possibilities for end states. For instance, when a compensation task fails, the termination criteria will be reached; i.e., no more transformation rules will be applicable, although the workflow is not in a desirable end state. In this case, manual intervention will be necessary to get workflow execution on the right track again.

Now the properties which a workflow model $\mathfrak{S}_1$ must satisfy in order to be sound can be expressed as: (i) *Proper termination*: the transition system terminates always resulting in one of the end states in $E^{\mathfrak{S}_1}$; (ii) *No dead tasks*: for each task X in $\mathfrak{S}_1$, the specification $\mathfrak{S}_0^X$ is one of the states in the transition system, where $\mathfrak{S}_0^X$ is an instance of $\mathfrak{S}_1$ in which a task instance x:X is annotated with <E>.

It is straightforward prove that for each workflow model $\mathfrak{S}_1$ the transition system (described by the rules in Tables 3 and 4) starting from the start state $\mathfrak{S}_0^s$, will terminate in one of the end states in $E^{\mathfrak{S}_1}$. In particular, given the start state and the transition system, we can construct all possible sequences of transformation rule applications by applying all transformation rules in all possible sequences, and inspect the resulting target specifications (those which cannot be transformed anymore) to check whether they are normal or compensation end states. In this way we "calculate" the state space, and prove that each path will eventually end in one of the end states. In addition to the soundness property, user-defined properties could be defined in the same format as above, i.e., by requiring that there exists a state in the transition system which has a certain feature. That is, we can define other properties as target instances (in other words states) and inspect the transition system (state space) to see whether that particular instance (state) exists.

4   Related Work

Kindler [14] advocated MDE, particularly the *Model-driven Architecture* (MDA) [18] for Process-Aware Information Systems (PAIS). Similar to our motivation, he also argues for the suitability of MDE in PAIS, however, although many of the MDE concepts are explained and put in relation to PAIS, a specific modelling language for workflow (or business) process modelling is not proposed.

Brüning et al. [6] present a strict metamodelling approach to workflow modelling, which makes it possible to easily express semantics of sophisticated transition relationships between activities using UML class diagrams and OCL constraints. Due to shortcomings of UML and OCL w.r.t. constraint evaluation combined with multi-level metamodelling, this approach flattens the three levels – metamodel, model and instance – into two levels. OCL constraints are defined at the metamodel level and they are enforced at the model/instance level. Our approach allows multi-level metamodelling with a unification of structural and OCL constraints into one formalism, and clearly distinguishes between the different levels of the metamodelling hierarchy.

Ghamarian et al. [13] employ a graph transformations-based framework, GROOVE, to provide semantics to behavioural models. Our approach extends graph transformations by using constraint-aware model transformations – i.e., considering diagrammatic constraints in transformation rule definitions and applications – which facilitate the definition of more fine grained rules and better control of their applications [26].

Wong et al. [28] present a semantics for a subset of BPMN in CSP and facilitate the use of model checkers like FDR for model verification. We are working on the model verification for our approach; more details can be found in Section 5.

There are several works that formalise compensation using process calculi, including *compensating* CSP (cCSP) [7] and *Sagas calculi* [5]. Chen et al. [8] further extend cCSP with semantic theory of failures and divergences of LRTs. In particular, they add non-deterministic choices, synchronization among parallel processes, hiding and recursion so as to provide support for compositional design and verification of LRTs by refinement and decomposition. These works provide solid theoretical foundations for compensation primitives and flow compositions. We will investigate these compositional features and include them in our future work.

Aït-Sadoune et al. [3] use the Event B method for formal description, modelling and validation of web services compositions. The approach suggests a refinement based method that encodes the BPEL models decompositions and formalises relevant properties as Event B properties which later can be proved. This work is not based on the MDE methodology which is necessary to have executable code automatically generated.

Damas et al. [9] extend high-level Message Sequence Charts with guards and compile the input models into an intermediate event-based formalism, the guarded Labeled Transition Systems. They propose tool-supported analysis techniques including model checking against state-based properties, state invariant generation, and guard analysis.

NOVA Workflow [22] is a framework for compensable workflow modeling which supports the modeling, execution and verification of workflow systems. It was extended by a domain specific language, $T_\square$, to support applications such as health services delivery [23]. However, it does not follow the metamodelling approach described here and may lead to impaired links between the workflow model and the generated code.

5   Conclusion and Future Work

This paper outlines a formal approach to compensable workflow modelling following MDE-methodologies and formal modelling principles. The approach provides a visually appealing technique for workflow modelling. Two different modelling formalisms are described: the first is used for the specification of workflow models while the second is used for the specification of their instances. Creation of instances is equivalent to creation of states (static semantics) while creation of sequences of transformation rule applications is equivalent to creation of execution paths (dynamic semantics). The presented modelling formalism is extended with new types, predicates and transformation rules to support compensation. This illustrates the flexibility of the MDE-based approach to extend modelling formalisms to support new behaviour. In addition, we use a metamodelling approach to define modelling languages facilitating the definition of different abstraction levels suitable for different users. In this way we may abstract away from formal details and overcome the complexity related to the use of formal methods.

We are using model checking (work in progress) to formally verify whether our workflow models fulfil desired properties. Currently we have an automated translator from workflow models to DVE (the modelling language for the DiVinE model checker), to let us verify LTL properties. As a proof of concept, the workflow modelling formalism and the automated translator are implemented as plugins to the DPF Workbench [15]. We are also developing an interface so the non-specialist can easily input LTL formulas for verification. This interface will allow the definition of requirements such as those on page 199 in a user-friendly syntax. Furthermore, we will investigate the theory of failures and divergences of LRTs which are elaborated in [8].

In future we plan to generate executable code to run real-life workflow software for application to healthcare and other safety critical systems. It is anticipated that the high overhead of the modelling formalism will be substantially offset by the benefits of automated generation of executable, verified code which is easily modified and accurately reflects the specifications of the processes modelled using the formalism.

Acknowledgements. This research is sponsored by Natural Sciences and Engineering Research Council of Canada and by the Atlantic Canada Opportunities Agency. Thanks to the anonymous reviewers who have contributed positively to the quality of the paper.

References

1. van der Aalst, W.M.P., van Hee, K.: Workflow Management: Models, Methods, and Systems. MIT Press (2002)
2. van der Aalst, W.M.P., ter Hofstede, A.H.M.: YAWL: Yet Another Workflow Language. Information Systems 30(4), 245–275 (2005)
3. Ait-Sadoune, I., Ait-Ameur, Y.: Stepwise Design of BPEL Web Services Compositions: An Event_B Refinement Based Approach. In: Lee, R., Ormandjieva, O., Abran, A., Constantinides, C. (eds.) SERA 2010. SCI, vol. 296, pp. 51–68. Springer, Heidelberg (2010)
4. Barr, M., Wells, C.: Category Theory for Computing Science, 2nd edn. Prentice Hall (1995)
5. Bruni, R., Melgratti, H., Montanari, U.: Theoretical Foundations for Compensations in Flow Composition Languages. In: POPL 2005, pp. 209–220. ACM (2005)

6. Brüning, J., Gogolla, M., Forbrig, P.: Modeling and Formally Checking Workflow Properties Using UML and OCL. In: Forbrig, P., Günther, H. (eds.) BIR 2010. LNBIP, vol. 64, pp. 130–145. Springer, Heidelberg (2010)

7. Butler, M., Hoare, T., Ferreira, C.: A trace semantics for long-running transactions. In: Abdallah, A.E., Jones, C.B., Sanders, J.W. (eds.) CSP25. LNCS, vol. 3525, pp. 133–150. Springer, Heidelberg (2005)

8. Chen, Z., Liu, Z., Wang, J.: Failure-Divergence Semantics and Refinement of Long Running Transactions. Theoretical Computer Science (to appear)

9. Damas, C., Lambeau, B., Roucoux, F., van Lamsweerde, A.: Analyzing critical process models through behavior model synthesis. In: ICSE 2009, pp. 441–451. IEEE Computer Society (2009)

10. Diskin, Z.: Mathematics of Generic Specifications for Model Management I and II. In: Encyclopedia of Database Technologies and Applications, pp. 351–366. Information Science Reference (2005)

11. Diskin, Z., Kadish, B., Piessens, F., Johnson, M.: Universal Arrow Foundations for Visual Modeling. In: Anderson, M., Cheng, P., Haarslev, V. (eds.) Diagrams 2000. LNCS (LNAI), vol. 1889, pp. 345–360. Springer, Heidelberg (2000)

12. Ehrig, H., Ehrig, K., Prange, U., Taentzer, G.: Fundamentals of Algebraic Graph Transformation. Springer (March 2006)

13. Ghamarian, A., de Mol, M., Rensink, A., Zambon, E., Zimakova, M.: Modelling and analysis using GROOVE. STTT, 1–26 (2011)

14. Kindler, E.: Model-based software engineering and process-aware information systems. In: Jensen, K., van der Aalst, W.M.P. (eds.) ToPNoC II. LNCS, vol. 5460, pp. 27–45. Springer, Heidelberg (2009)

15. Lamo, Y., Wang, X., Mantz, F., MacCaull, W., Rutle, A.: DPF Workbench: A Diagrammatic Multi-Layer Domain Specific (Meta-)Modelling Environment. In: Lee, R. (ed.) Computer and Information Science 2012. SCI, vol. 429, pp. 37–52. Springer, Heidelberg (2012)

16. Lapadula, A., Pugliese, R., Tiezzi, F.: Specifying and Analysing SOC Applications with COWS. In: Degano, P., De Nicola, R., Meseguer, J. (eds.) Concurrency, Graphs and Models. LNCS, vol. 5065, pp. 701–720. Springer, Heidelberg (2008)

17. OASIS: Web services business process execution language version 2.0 (2007), http://docs.oasis-open.org/wsbpel/2.0/OS/wsbpel-v2.0-OS.html

18. Object Management Group: MDA Guide (June 2003), http://www.omg.org/cgi-bin/doc?omg/03-06-01

19. OMG: Business Process Model and Notation (BPMN) Version 2.0 (January 2011), http://www.omg.org/spec/BPMN/2.0/

20. Ottensooser, A., Fekete, A., Reijers, H.A., Mendling, J., Menictas, C.: Making sense of business process descriptions: An experimental comparison of graphical and textual notations. Journal of Systems and Software 85(3), 596–606 (2012)

21. Ouyang, C., Dumas, M., ter Hofstede, A.H.M., van der Aalst, W.M.P.: From BPMN Process Models to BPEL Web Services. In: ICWS, pp. 285–292. IEEE Computer Society (2006)

22. Rabbi, F.: Design, Development and Verification of a Compensable Workflow Modeling Language. Master's thesis, Dept. of Math, Stats and CS, StFX University, Canada (2011)

23. Rabbi, F., MacCaull, W.: $T_\square$: A Domain Specific Language for Rapid Workflow Development. In: France, R.B., Kazmeier, J., Breu, R., Atkinson, C. (eds.) MODELS 2012. LNCS, vol. 7590, pp. 36–52. Springer, Heidelberg (2012)

24. Rutle, A.: Diagram Predicate Framework: A Formal Approach to MDE. Ph.D. thesis, Department of Informatics, University of Bergen, Norway (2010)

25. Rutle, A., MacCaull, W., Wang, H., Lamo, Y.: A Metamodelling Approach to Behavioural Modelling. In: BM-FA 2012, pp. 5:1–5:10. ACM (2012)
26. Rutle, A., Rossini, A., Lamo, Y., Wolter, U.: A formal approach to the specification and transformation of constraints in MDE. JLAP 81(4), 422–457 (2012)
27. Wang, H., Rutle, A., MacCaull, W.: A Formal Diagrammatic Approach to Timed Workflow Modelling. In: TASE 2012, pp. 167–174. IEEE Computer Society (2012)
28. Wong, P.Y.H., Gibbons, J.: A Process Semantics for BPMN. In: Liu, S., Araki, K. (eds.) ICFEM 2008. LNCS, vol. 5256, pp. 355–374. Springer, Heidelberg (2008)

Towards Generic MDE Support for Extracting Purpose-Specific Healthcare Models from Annotated, Unstructured Texts

Pieter Van Gorp[1], Irene Vanderfeesten[1], Willem Dalinghaus[1],
Josh Mengerink[1], Bram van der Sanden[1], and Pieter Kubben[2]

[1] School of Industrial Engineering, Eindhoven University of Technology
`{p.m.e.v.gorp,i.t.p.vanderfeesten}@tue.nl`
[2] Department of Neurosurgery, Maastricht University Medical Center
`pieter@kubben.nl`

Abstract. Once healthcare-specific models have been captured formally (i.e., in a metamodel-based language), the application of model transformation, analysis and code generation techniques is rather straightforward. Unfortunately, in many healthcare settings valuable domain knowledge is hidden in unstructured text (e.g., in a research paper or a national report on clinical guidelines). This motivates the need for tools to annotate such texts with metadata. Such tools can be prototyped easily for one type of healthcare artifacts (e.g., for clinical guidelines or care pathways) and one purpose (e.g., for workflow management or decision support) but it is a research challenge to build a robust and generic (i.e., metamodel-independent) tool for this important type of model extraction support. This paper desribes our ongoing work to building such a tool on top of a state-of-the-art MDE platform.

1 Introduction

Governments, insurance organizations, hospital boards, physicians and patient organizations support the relevance of rigorous engineering methods for the development and certification of information systems in healthcare. Model-Driven Engineering (MDE) techniques are particularly strong at separating medical and organizational concepts from system implementation details. This is important since information system architectures vary significantly within and between care institutions while at the conceptual level patients cross the institutional and system boundaries. As in most other engineering disciplines, models in MDE are simplified representations that enable one to reason more easily about complex issues. The distinguishing factor is that MDE techniques can combine multiple modeling languages (and formalisms).

MDE leverages explicit modeling language definitions (called metamodels) and model transformation definitions to break down complex modeling problems in more manageable subproblems. We have recently demonstrated that MDE technology is particularly mature in support for generating powerful model

J. Weber and I. Perseil (Eds.): FHIES 2012, LNCS 7789, pp. 213–221, 2013.
© Springer-Verlag Berlin Heidelberg 2013

editors from annotated metamodels [1]. This short paper focuses on providing novel support for extracting models from unstructured texts.

The remainder of this paper is structured as follows: Section 2 presents a typical example of a clinical decision support (CDS) system. Section 3 presents our solution in two steps (first specific to the CDS example and then more generally). Section 4 describes related and future work and Section 5 concludes.

2   Example Clinical Decision Support System

Fig. 1 shows a clinical guideline (CG) supported by the Congress of Neurological Surgeons and the American Association of Neurological Surgeons. The selected guideline is that for surgical management of depressed cranial fractures.

> **RECOMMENDATIONS**
> (see *Methodology*)
>
> **Indications**
> - Patients with open (compound) cranial fractures depressed greater than the thickness of the cranium should undergo operative intervention to prevent infection.
> - Patients with open (compound) depressed cranial fractures may be treated nonoperatively if there is no clinical or radiographic evidence of dural penetration, significant intracranial hematoma, depression greater than 1 cm, frontal sinus involvement, gross cosmetic deformity, wound infection, pneumocephalus, or gross wound contamination.
> - Nonoperative management of closed (simple) depressed cranial fractures is a treatment option.
>
> **Timing**
> - Early operation is recommended to reduce the incidence of infection.
>
> **Methods**
> - Elevation and debridement is recommended as the surgical method of choice.
> - Primary bone fragment replacement is a surgical option in the absence of wound infection at the time of surgery.
> - All management strategies for open (compound) depressed fractures should include antibiotics.
>
> KEY WORDS: Antibiotic prophylaxis, Burr hole, Cranial fracture, Craniotomy, Depressed cranial fracture, Depressed skull fracture, Head injury, Skull fracture, Surgical technique, Traumatic brain injury

Fig. 1. Example of a Clinical Guideline recommendation (summary based on [2])

As a concrete example of a CDS system derived from such a guideline, consider Fig. 2. That figure shows screenshots of an app that enables specialists to (1) lookup a guideline from a catalogue and (2) retrieve recommendations by entering patient-specific information. Fig. 2(a) shows the app after selecting our example guideline. In our example scenario, the user answers respectively "yes", "no", "yes" (cfr., the "on", "off", "on" buttons) on the series of questions shown on Fig. 2(a) to 2(c). According to the guideline, this leads to the suggestion that there is evidence in favor of performing an early operation (Fig. 2(d)). The underlying decision algorithm is not directly visible in the guideline text. Some medical papers do provide flowcharts to make the proposed decision making process more explicit. However, specialists in a concrete care facility typically still have to adapt such flowcharts to their specific situation. This paper starts from our collaboration with a Dutch academic hospital.

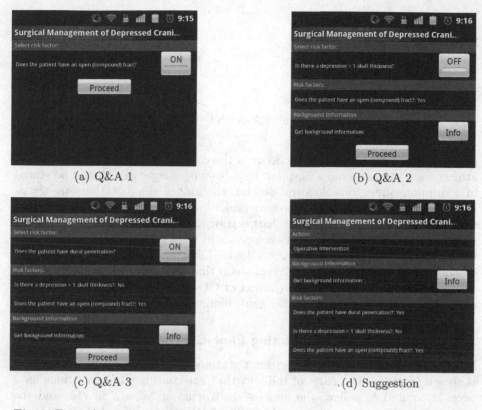

(a) Q&A 1   (b) Q&A 2

(c) Q&A 3   (d) Suggestion

Fig. 2. Example execution of the generated app running on an Android smartphone

In this hospital, one of the neurosurgeons maintains a set of flowcharts to formalize a set of specialized guidelines. The neurosurgeon also programs CDS support in apps such as the one from Fig. 2. These apps are quite popular in both the Android and iOS app stores [3]. Remarkably, the flowcharts are just informal documentation for these apps. We observed that by using MDE techniques, the apps could be generated automatically. That could reduce the development effort and the risk for inconsistencies. It would require however the use of a flowchart editor with a custom metamodel (e.g., with support for modeling CDS questions and links back to medical evidence).

This paper focuses on a key limitation of MDE and our suggested way to overcome it. Our extended experience report also clarifies to Health IT practitioners what existing MDE tools can offer them in the first place [1].

3   Deriving Models from Annotated, Unstructured Text

Fig. 3 sketches our proposed tool-chain from an end-user perspective: first, medical specialists annotate scientific CGs. This can happen in the context of their

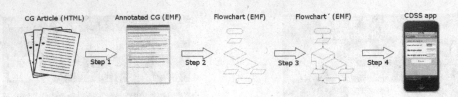

Fig. 3. Model-driven, evidence-based, development of CDS apps

personal continuous learning process or in the context of regularly planned literature review cycles within a hospital. In this step, annotations should be stored in a computer-interpretable form. Second, the guideline annotations are transformed automatically into a flowchart skeleton model. Third, the flowchart is manually refined. Finally, the flowchart is transformed automatically into a CDS app. Configuration files for a more heavyweight CDS system could be generated too but this is not implemented at the time of writing. In the following, we first demonstrate a metamodel-specific tool-chain that we have used to better understand the above workflow in the context of CG-based CDS. Then, we describe our ongoing efforts to derive similar tool-chains more efficiently in the large.

3.1   Ad-Hoc Support: Extracting Flow-Charts from CGs

Fig. 5 shows the text from Fig. 1 within the annotation tool. The title annotation is shown in green. The parts of the text that are considered observations have been annotated in yellow, the actions/treatments are shown in red, and the explanatory elements are shown in blue. The bottom left of Fig. 1 shows controls for creating new annotations while the top left shows a tree preview of the guideline model that is under construction. By clicking the *compile* button, this representation is translated into a metamodel-based flowchart model (step 2 from Fig. 3), which can be refined manually (step 3 from Fig. 3). Fig. 4 shows a screenshot of an example use of this editor. The left pane shows the editor palette, which enables the instantiation of the concepts from the syntax defintion. The middle pane shows an example flowchart diagram. In the screenshot, the "Hematoma" node from the upper left is selected and its details are shown in the rightmost editor pane. The pane enables a.o. associating reference papers (i.e., evidence) to the node. The editor instantiates models in such a format that they can be seemlessly processed by other special purpose MDE tools (e.g., for transformation and verification, see http://www.eclipse.org/modeling/).

We have also developed a prototypical code generator for realizing step 4 from Fig. 3. The complete tool-chain prototype was implemented by two junior programmers with basic Java programming skills. Students did receive guidance by one MDE expert, primarily in the use of the Epsilon framework [4]. Epsilon's Eugenia component has saved valuable time during the development of the CDS-specific flowchart model editor (shown in Fig. 4). The annotation editor (shown in Fig. 5) as well as its simple *"annotation to model compiler"* have been hand-crafted.

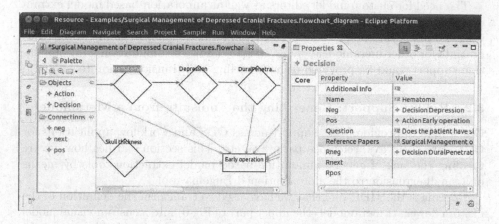

Fig. 4. Example Use of the MDE-based Clinical Guideline Editor Prototype

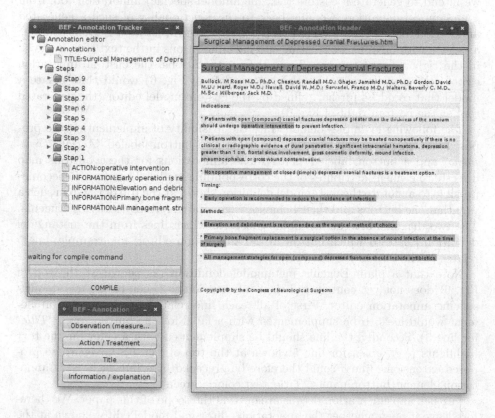

Fig. 5. Demonstration of support for elicitating model elements using text annotations

The need for custom model editors as well as annotation-based model extractors goes far beyond CGs and CDS, as discussed further in our related and future work section. Therefore, instead of replicating functionality in hand-crafted components for other metamodels, we investigated how the annotation and compilation support could be provided using modeling and transformation techniques.

3.2   Robust Support: Generating the Toolsuite from a Metamodel

Our aim is to provide MDE support across CDS and workflow applications for CGs, care pathways, reference pathways, etc. This section clarifies how we are tackling the lack of generic annotation-based model extraction tools by means of a small extension to the aforementioned Eugenia tool.

Eugenia is the MDE tool that we have used to transform the definition of the custom flowchart metamodel (the upper part of Fig 6) into a custom visual model editor. That existing Eugenia functionality is visualized by the bold arrow in the right part of Fig 6. The bold arrow in the left part of the figure represents the proposed new functionality for the Epsilon platform. That arrow visualizes how we intend to generate a custom (i.e., metamodel-specific) annotation tool from a metamodel definition. Coming back to the functionality of such a generated annotation tool: the left part of Fig. 6's *"Generated Annotation Editor"* contains a palette with buttons for creating specific annotations in the text that is shown in the right part of the box. From these annotations, the custom annotation editor (the generated tool at the bottom left of Fig. 6) would then create a model that could be further refined by the custom model editor (the generated tool at the bottom right of Fig. 6).

The following examples demonstrate the feasibility of implementing the proposed Eugenia extensions: the palette contains a button labeled *"Action/Treatment"* and a button labeled *"Title"*. The annotations for these buttons map directly to element attributes of the corresponding model. Therefore, it becomes possible to annotate the metamodel definition shown at the top of Fig. 6 in such a way that the buttons and their behavior is generated automatically by Eugenia. The two diagonal arcs on the figure illustrate which lines from the metamodel definition relate to which button in the annotation editor: for example, line 5 relates to the button labeled *"Title"*.

Note that a plain Eugenia metamodel definition (as shown at the top of Fig. 6) does not yet contain sufficient information to generate the metamodel-specific annotation editor. First of all, each line related to an annotation element would have to be supplemented with a label for the button (e.g., *"Title"* for line 5). Secondly, the line should be supplemented with a color for the text highlights (e.g., *green* for line 5 shown at the top of Fig. 6). Given these proposed extensions, line 5 could therefore be preceded by a line such as: "@annotation.element(button.name='Title',text.color='green')".

Further implementation details are outside the scope of this paper. We therefore leave it open whether the annotation editor and model editor shown at the bottom of Fig. 6 are separate tools or one integrated component. Regardless, generic model transformation languages/tools could be used to automatically

Eugenia Metamodel Definition

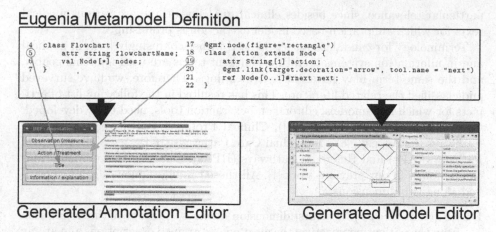

```
 4   class Flowchart {                     17   @gmf.node(figure="rectangle")
 5       attr String flowchartName;        18   class Action extends Node {
 6       val Node[*] nodes;                19       attr String[1] action;
 7   }                                     20       @gmf.link(target.decoration="arrow", tool.name = "next")
                                           21       ref Node[0..1]#rnext next;
                                           22   }
```

Generated Annotation Editor   **Generated Model Editor**

Fig. 6. Generating annotation tools from an extended Eugenia metamodel

produce and optimize output models. For the sake of persistence and consistency, we propose that the complete texts as well as the begin and end indices of annotations are stored also inside the metamodel-based output model.

4   Related and Future Work

We evaluated tool support for systematically deriving clinical guideline models from medical literature. We focussed on MDE tools since these are known to excel in the linkage of models with different purposes and at various levels of abstraction. MDE tools are also known to support the co-evolution of conceptual models with derived software systems. To the best of our knowledge, there are no experience reports on the linkage of MDE artifacts with unstructured documents.

Some isolated engineering efforts have been published outside the MDE context. For example, Lobach et al. [5] describe a conceptual process for translating informal guidelines into computer-interpretable representations. Concerning tool support, the Yale Center for Medical Informatics has developed and evaluated GEM Cutter II [6]. From the evaluation perspective, the Yale group has demonstrated that *an annotation-based approach to guideline model extraction is promising*, but also that *additional analysis is needed to determine the feasibility of offering "GEM-cut" recommendations nationally* (in the US). From the tooling point of view, we observe that GEM Cutter (1) is based directly on XML technologies rather than on formal metamodels, (2) does not provide support for visual models and (3) implicitly imposes one particular metamodel. We aim at tool support that excels on these three points: (1) we aim at an annotation-based model extraction infrastructure based on Eclipse ECore and EMF, which are the industry-standards for metamodeling in MDE; (2) we aim at supporting visual models, especially since medical papers often include flowchart based summaries; and (3) we aim at adaptable metamodels. We consider the last point of particular relevance, since besides clinical guidelines there are various medical texts for which annotation-based model extraction is promising.

Terminology for candidate *models* is used rather confusingly both in medical and in information systems literature: different terms are used interchangeably, and the same term may have different meanings. Therefore, we have surveyed and classified the related literature. This has resulted in the following list of artifacts for which metamodels, editors, and extraction tools, need to be developed: Clinical Guidelines (CGs, e.g., [2]), Clinical Protocols (CPRs, e.g., [7]), Care Pathways (CPAs, e.g., [8]), Individual Care Pathways (ICPs, e.g., [9]), Assigned Pathways (APs) and Reference Pathways (RPAs). Our summarized definitions can be found in our previous work [1]. All these candidate models can be classified along two dimensions:

D1 (Patient Scope). The first dimension involves the scope of the description from the patient perspective: the most coarse grained descriptions aim at any type of patient, regardless of care groups. Other descriptions aim at multiple patients but within one specific care group. Finally, some descriptions are specific to an individual patient.

D2 (Provider Scope). In the provider aggregation dimension, some descriptions aim at multiple organizations while others are oriented at only one specific care organization.

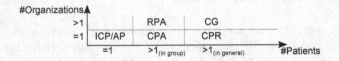

Fig. 7. 2D Classification of Process Oriented Care Descriptions

Fig. 7 shows that the classification of the aforementioned care descriptions in the proposed 2-dimensional space: when referring to the concrete goals and activities for one patient within one organization ($=1$, $=1$), one is considering ICPs and APs. When referring to the process descriptions for a group of patients within one organization ($> 1_{in\,group}$, $=1$), one is considering CPAs. When for such a group of patients one is referring to an abstract process description that is shared by multiple organizations ($> 1_{in\,group}$, >1) then one is considering RPAs. In the context of decision support for patients regardless of groups, CPRs are descriptions used within organizational boundaries ($> 1_{in\,general}$, $=1$) while CGs are used beyond these boundaries ($> 1_{in\,general}$, >1). All these artifacts are semantically related and since they can also evolve over time, our classification opens interesting opportunities for applying MDE techniques for co-evolution (e.g., those from Cichetti et al. [10]) in a challenging healthcare setting. In combination with our various metamodel-specific annotation tools, the traceability to related textual artifacts becomes manageable too. The practical integration of these techniques is the subject of our future work.

5   Conclusions

This short paper focuses on a specific MDE contribution: the development of a CDS based on the extraction of models from unstructured clinical guideline texts. However, our line of work is at the interface between Health Informatics and MDE research. Within the paradigm of using light-weight, custom editors instead of using heavyweight *"one size fits all"* editors (e.g., editors based on GEM, GLIF or SAGE), we have identified the lack of tools to extract purpose-specific models from unstructured texts. Besides presenting an exploratory, ad-hoc implementation of such a CDS-specific model extraction tool, we have discussed how a state-of-the-art MDE toolsuite can be extended for generating similar extraction tools in the large. Generating such tools is important since they are needed for a variety of healthcare and purpose-specific metamodels.

References

1. Van Gorp, P., Vanderfeesten, I., Dalinghaus, W., Mengerink, J., van der Sanden, B., Kubben, P.: MDE support for process-oriented health information systems: from theory to practice. In: Pre-proceedings of FHIES 2012 (August 2012)
2. Ross Bullock, M., et al.: Surgical management of depressed cranial fractures. Neurosurgery 58(suppl. 3), S56–S60, discussion Si–iv (2006)
3. Kubben, P.: Neuromind (December 2012),
   http://apps.digitalneurosurgeon.com/neuromind
4. Kolovos, D.S., Rose, L.M., Abid, S.B., Paige, R.F., Polack, F.A.C., Botterweck, G.: Taming EMF and GMF using model transformation. In: Petriu, D.C., Rouquette, N., Haugen, Ø. (eds.) MODELS 2010, Part I. LNCS, vol. 6394, pp. 211–225. Springer, Heidelberg (2010)
5. Lobach, D.F., Kerner, N.: A systematic process for converting text-based guidelines into a linear algorithm for electronic implementation. In: Proc. AMIA Symp., pp. 507–511 (2000)
6. Haskell, L.T., Monteforte, P.M.J., Shiffman, R.N., Coates, V.H., Nix, M.P.: S92 – applying the Guideline Elements Model (GEM) cutter II tool to guidelines represented in the national guideline clearinghouse (www.guideline.gov). Otolaryngol. Head Neck Surg. 143(suppl. 60-61) (July 2010)
7. Lorne Community Hospital: Anaphylaxis (2007),
   http://www.health.vic.gov.au/qum/downloads/anaphylaxis.pdf
8. South East Wales Cardiac Network: Integrated care pathway cardiac rehabilitation (May 2005), http://www.wales.nhs.uk/sitesplus/documents/986/ICPCardiacRehabPathwayJan2006.pdf
9. Elm Mount Units: Individual recovery/care plan review elm mount units (August 2012), http://www.mhcirl.ie/Inspectorate_of_Mental_Health_Services/ICPT/Elm%20Mount_CPT.pdf
10. Cicchetti, A., Di Ruscio, D., Eramo, R., Pierantonio, A.: Automating co-evolution in model-driven engineering. In: Proceedings of the 2008 12th International IEEE Enterprise Distributed Object Computing Conference, EDOC 2008, pp. 222–231. IEEE Computer Society, Washington, DC (2008)

Author Index